The Quick & Easy Paleo Cookbook

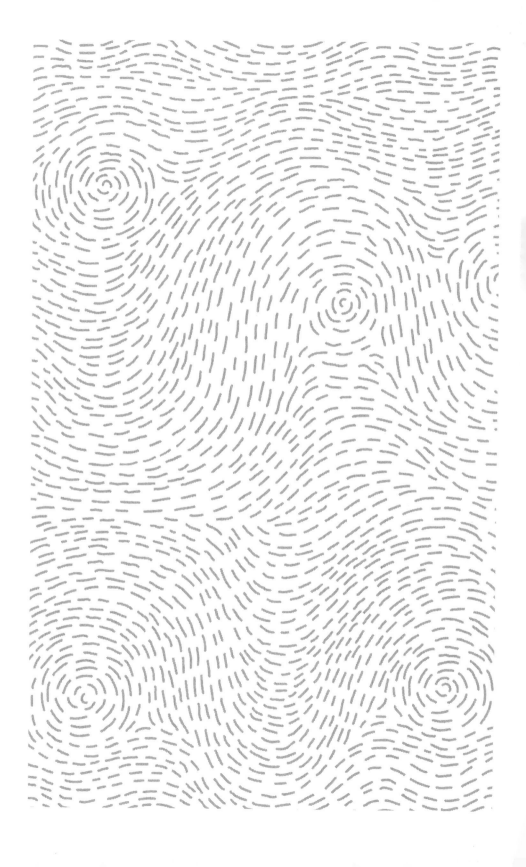

The Quick & Easy Paleo Cookbook

77 PALEO DIET RECIPES MADE IN MINUTES

TELAMON
PRESS

For general information on our other products and services or to obtain technical support, please contact our Customer Care Department within the United States at (866) 744-2665, or outside the United States at (510) 253-0500.

Telamon Press publishes its books in a variety of electronic and print formats. Some content that appears in print may not be available in electronic books, and vice versa.

TRADEMARKS: Telamon Press and the Telamon Press logo are trademarks or registered trademarks of Callisto Media Inc. and/or its affiliates, in the United States and other countries, and may not be used without written permission. All other trademarks are the property of their respective owners. Telamon Press is not associated with any product or vendor mentioned in this book.

ISBN: Print 978-1-62315-345-8| eBook 978-1-62315-346-5

Contents

Introduction

Welcome to *The Quick & Easy Paleo Cookbook*. Whether you've picked up this book because you want to lose weight, or you simply want to feel better, you've come to the right place. The Paleo diet offers these benefits and more.

The Paleo diet is based on the idea that our bodies, which evolved over millions of years to ingest a hunter-gatherer diet, simply can't tolerate the modern diet's low-nutrient, highly refined carbohydrates and toxic chemicals. By eating in a way that mimics the way our ancestors ate before the agricultural and industrial revolutions, Paleo diet followers hope to optimize their health while minimizing the risk of chronic disease. In the process, many find that they also experience other benefits:

- Weight loss
- Clearer skin and elimination of skin conditions like eczema
- Lowered blood pressure and reduced symptoms of chronic illnesses such as type 2 diabetes, rheumatoid arthritis, and celiac disease
- Reduced allergic reactions
- Elimination of bothersome digestive symptoms such as gas, bloating, diarrhea, and constipation

The Quick & Easy Paleo Cookbook is filled with information that will help you incorporate the Paleo diet into your life with ease. You will gain a full understanding of the theory behind the Paleo diet and you'll have the information you need to adopt the diet yourself.

While many Paleo cookbooks and websites rely on complicated or time-consuming cooking techniques and expensive or hard-to-find ingredients, this book provides recipes that are, as the title states, quick and easy to make, and that use ingredients that are both affordable and commonly available. And all the recipes in the book can be prepared in 30 minutes or less.

The book is divided into two parts. Part One provides you with all the basics of the Paleo diet. It examines the Paleo way of eating and the related health benefits. It also provides a detailed guide to getting started on the Paleo diet, including lists of which foods to eat and which to avoid, and advice on meal planning, stocking your pantry, and cooking quick and delicious meals that adhere to the plan.

Part Two offers seventy-seven quick and easy recipes that follow the Paleo diet guidelines. These dishes are a cinch to make, highly nutritious, and full of flavor. With these recipes in hand, you'll begin your Paleo diet eating delicious and satisfying meals.

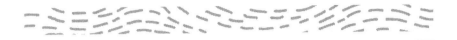

PART ONE

Getting Started

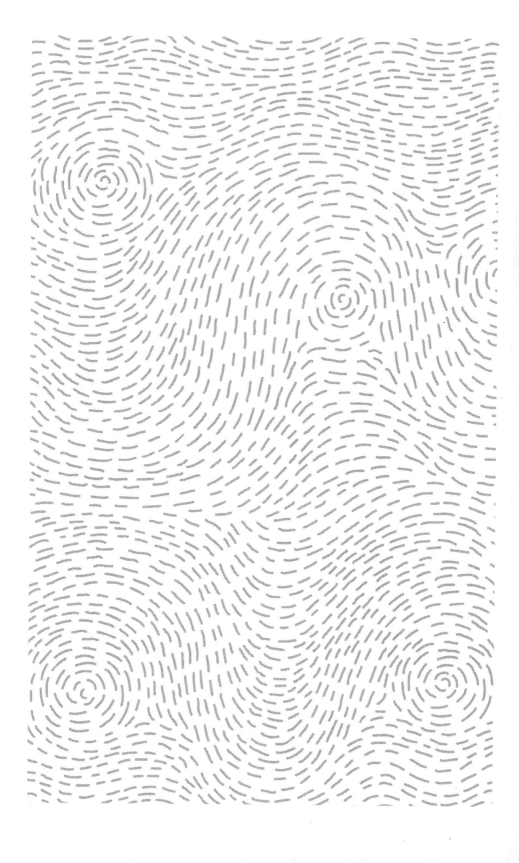

CHAPTER ONE

The Basics of the Paleo Diet

In its most basic terms, the Paleo diet is a diet that mimics the eating habits of our ancestors. This means a diet consisting of whole, minimally processed foods that could have been gathered or hunted in our ancestors' immediate environs.

While it's true that to adopt the Paleo diet, you'll need to overhaul the way you eat and think about food, this book will make it easy. It tells you everything you need to know to get started and to incorporate the diet's principles into your daily life.

WHAT IS THE PALEO DIET?

Often referred to as the caveman diet, primal diet, or Paleolithic diet, the Paleo diet resembles the eating habits of the early humans who populated Earth. These people didn't have agriculture. They didn't cultivate crops or mill grains. They didn't eat refined sugars, grains, dairy, oils, or any of the highly processed foods that are so common today. And so they probably did not suffer from modern-day diseases like type 2 diabetes, obesity, and cardiovascular disease.

These early humans subsisted on a diet made up of whatever foods they could find in their natural environment: free-range meats, fish, nuts, seeds, fruits, and vegetables. In other words, they ate unprocessed, seasonal, local, organic, whole foods.

But around ten thousand years ago, many humans settled in groups—for support, companionship, safety, and other reasons—and they began to cultivate vegetables and domesticate animals for their food. These people were no longer wandering the land in search of their next meal. They became more sedentary, and learned to refine grains and other foods in order to have a predictable, easily accessible, and convenient source of nutrition.

The downside of all this newfound convenience is that the changes in the human diet, combined with reduced physical activity, have caused us to become increasingly overweight and plagued by diseases. The theory behind the Paleo diet is that we humans simply haven't adapted to eating all of these highly processed foods. These processed foods, Paleo proponents assert, cause inflammation at the cellular level, promoting disease.

So the premise of the Paleo diet is that if we could go back to eating the way our predecessors did, we might be able to cure ourselves of the modern diseases that plague us. The Paleo diet, then, involves eating the types of foods the early people ate. This means that we should avoid any foods that cannot be obtained without farming, domesticating animals, or high-tech processing—like grains, legumes, refined sugar, dairy products, processed oils, and chemical additives.

You may be thinking: Wait, doesn't that cover just about everything? It's true that the modern diet relies heavily on processed grains, sugars, dairy, vegetable oils, and other non-Paleo foods. But there is a world of natural, delicious foods that are available to the Paleo dieter: fresh, whole foods. Meats, seafood, eggs, vegetables, fruit, healthy fats, nuts, and seeds are all on the Paleo menu. Another way to remember the basic parameters of the diet is: Eat plants and animals, essentially as they are found in nature.

By following the Paleo diet, you will be eating fresh, healthy, nutrient-packed foods that have been prepared in ways that maintain their healthful qualities. And you will likely find that you feel better than ever because you are eating foods that support your body rather than sabotage it.

BENEFITS OF THE PALEO DIET

Because the Paleo diet is based on eating whole, natural, organic foods, there are many benefits to the diet.

Reduced Risk of Disease

There's no denying that more and more people suffer from modern diseases such as obesity, high blood pressure, diabetes, heart disease, stroke, and autoimmune diseases. Some scientists believe that this rise in "diseases of affluence" is caused by the fact that we consume carbohydrates in the form of grains, sugar, and starchy vegetables, and that these items can harm the mucous membranes in the digestive system, making it possible for harmful substances to enter the bloodstream. This then causes an immune response that, if it becomes chronic, can cause disease. Furthermore, eating carbohydrates can lead to spikes in blood sugar that, over a period of time, can eventually lead to insulin resistance, diabetes, and the development of metabolic disease.

Get More Nutrients, Not Less

A common misconception about the Paleo diet is that it is high in protein and fat, and low in other nutrients. The truth is that by eliminating high-calorie, low-nutrient carbohydrates and other processed foods from your diet, you will automatically begin to eat more nutrient-dense vegetables, healthy fats, nuts, seeds, and fruit. These foods are loaded with vitamins and minerals. In fact, a strict Paleo diet of meats, seafood, vegetables, and fruits provides all of the nutrients you need. And because of the improved digestive function and decreased systemic inflammation you'll enjoy as a result of the Paleo diet, you'll be absorbing a much higher percentage of the nutrients in the foods you eat.

Control Blood Sugar

Refined sugars wreak havoc with your blood glucose levels and can ultimately make you overweight, tired, and cranky. Even artificial sweeteners pose problems. Removing refined sugar and artificial sweeteners from your diet will help you feel better, lose weight, and reduce your risk of disease. Also, following a diet rich in lean protein and high-fiber plant foods will help control your blood sugar, thereby preventing weight gain and type 2 diabetes.

Weight Loss

Although weight loss isn't always the primary reason that people choose the Paleo diet, most Paleo dieters do drop pounds, as the result of improved metabolic processes and digestive health, better sleep, stress management, and proper quantities of vitamins, minerals, and healthy fats.

Improved Digestion

Because the Paleo diet is high in fiber, it reduces bloat and improves the gut flora that contribute to healthy digestion. Most Paleo dieters experience a drastic reduction in digestive symptoms such as gas, bloating, diarrhea, and constipation.

FOODS TO AVOID AND FOODS TO ENJOY

At the most basic level, eating Paleo means eating vegetables, fruits, meats, fish, healthy fats, nuts, and seeds, and avoiding grains, foods made from grains (breads, pastas, rice, etc.), beans and legumes (including peanuts, soy, and foods made from them), dairy, certain vegetable oils, refined sugars, and artificial additives.

The Problem with Grains

Grains are full of lectins, sugar-binding proteins that are found in the seeds of plants. The purpose of lectins is to protect the seeds so that they can reproduce. They do this by causing intestinal distress (diarrhea, nausea, bloating, vomiting, even death) to any animal that consumes them in quantity in order to discourage them from coming back for more.

Lectins attack the intestinal lining, wreaking havoc on the digestive system. They destroy cells and compromise intestinal villi, thereby reducing the body's ability to absorb nutrients. They have even been shown to contribute to the prediabetic condition called leptin resistance, which contributes to obesity.

Lectins can even create holes in the intestinal lining, leading to a condition called "leaky gut syndrome," which then allow food particles, toxins, and lectins themselves into the bloodstream. There they bind to tissue (kidneys, liver, pancreas, etc.), causing an immune response wherein the body attacks otherwise healthy tissue and innocuous food particles. This is how food sensitivities are created, and it can cause everything from migraine headaches to eczema, weight gain, and depression. It can also contribute to serious autoimmune disorders such as Crohn's disease, irritable bowel syndrome, celiac disease, lupus, multiple sclerosis, and rheumatoid arthritis.

Refined Sugar and Artificial Sweeteners

Refined sugar is avoided on the Paleo diet for several reasons. First, refined sugar is simply not nutritious. It is high in calories, but devoid of minerals, vitamins, fiber, protein, and other nutrients that help your body function.

Furthermore, eating excess sugar causes erratic blood glucose levels, which can lead to sugar addiction, insulin resistance, weight gain, obesity, metabolic syndrome, prediabetes, type 2 diabetes, polycystic ovarian syndrome, and many other problems.

Sugar also suppresses the immune system and can cause fructose malabsorption, a condition in which unabsorbed fructose remains in your digestive tract where it feeds gut bacteria, causing gas, bloating, diarrhea or constipation, and abdominal pain. This malabsorption can lead to a host of ailments, including malnutrition and depression.

Beans and Legumes

Beans and legumes are also avoided on the Paleo diet. They're high in lectins and other anti-nutrients like phytic acid, which binds to the minerals magnesium, calcium, zinc, and iron in your gut and prevents them from being absorbed by your body. Paleo proponents believe that eating legumes can lead to gastrointestinal issues, autoimmune reactions, and nutrient deficiency.

Exceptions to the no-legumes rule are green legumes encapsulated in pods, like green beans, string beans, green peas, snap peas, and snow peas. While these legumes do contain phytic acids and lectins, they have them in reduced quantity. The greener a plant is, the lower the level of phytic acid and lectins it contains. You'd have to eat a whole lot of these green veggies to ingest enough anti-nutrients to do any real damage.

Vegetable and Seed Oils

Vegetable and seed oils—soybean, canola, corn, peanut, cottonseed, safflower, and sunflower—are high in easily oxidized polyunsaturated fatty acids (PUFAs) and pro-inflammatory omega-6 fatty acids. Oxidation decreases the oil's nutritional value and produces free radicals, which can attack and damage your body's cells, cause systemic inflammation, and increase your risk of chronic diseases. Consuming foods with excessive amounts of omega-6 fatty acids can also cause systemic inflammation and contribute to the development of disease and autoimmune conditions.

Dairy Products

Dairy products (milk, cream, cheese, butter) are extremely hard for the human digestive tract to digest. It's been estimated that as much as 80 percent of the world's population is lactose intolerant to some degree. The reason is that we are not genetically programmed to consume dairy after we're weaned, and we may not be programmed to consume cow's milk at all. Consuming dairy can cause major digestive problems, fatigue, and skin problems, and can prevent weight loss.

Paleo-Unfriendly Foods

By eliminating grains, legumes, vegetable oils, dairy, and other problematic foods, the Paleo diet can significantly reduce systemic inflammation and your risk of chronic diseases, including diabetes, heart attack, stroke, gastrointestinal ailments, autoimmune diseases, arthritis, and more. Following is a list of foods to avoid on the Paleo diet.

Grains

Amaranth

Buckwheat

Corn

Oats

Quinoa

Rice

Rye

Sorghum

Spelt

Wheat

Wild rice

Foods made from grains

Bagels

Bread

Cake

Cookies

Flour (wheat, corn, sorghum, rice, etc.)

Muffins

Pasta

Tortillas

Dairy

Butter

Cheese

Cottage cheese

Ghee

Kefir

Milk

Sour cream

Whey protein powders

Yogurt

Beans and legumes

Black beans

Garbanzo beans (chickpeas)

Lentils

Peanuts

Pinto beans

Red beans

Soy (including soy sauce, miso, tofu, and any other foods containing soy)

White beans

Vegetable oils

Any hydrogenated or partially
   hydrogenated oil
Canola oil
Corn oil
Cottonseed oil

Peanut oil
Safflower oil
Sesame oil
Soy oil
Sunflower oil

Refined sugars and artificial sweeteners

Corn syrup (and high-fructose
   corn syrup)
Equal (aspartame)
Fructose

Malt syrup
Splenda (sucralose)
Sugar

Paleo-Friendly Foods

While the list of foods you will give up in order to embrace a healthy Paleo lifestyle is long and might contain some of your favorites, there are countless wholesome, delicious, and extremely nutritious foods that you can enjoy on the Paleo diet. And eating them exclusively is virtually guaranteed to make you feel better than ever.

Vegetables

Almost all vegetables are Paleo-approved. Visit your local farmers' market to find some new favorites.

Beets
Cabbage
Chard, kale, and other dark,
   leafy greens
Carrots
Eggplants
Garlic
Green beans, peas, snow peas,
   snap peas
Lettuce

Mushrooms
Onions
Parsnips
Peppers
Radishes
Root vegetables (rutabaga, turnips, etc.)
Seaweed and other sea vegetables
Squash
Sweet potatoes*
Tomatoes

*Sweet potatoes, which are full of nutrients and high in fiber, are allowed on the Paleo diet, but white potatoes are controversial. Potatoes fit the parameters of allowed foods (they are a plant food that can be eaten raw or with minimal processing), but they are high in starch and calories and contain minimal nutrients. Most Paleo experts put white potatoes on their "avoid" list because they cause a blood glucose spike.

Fruits

Buy local, seasonal, organically grown fruits whenever you can. If you are trying to lose weight, you may want to limit your fruit intake to just a serving or two a day, since many fruits are high in natural sugars and, therefore, calories.

Apples	Mangos
Apricots	Melon
Bananas	Nectarines
Berries	Peaches
Cherries	Papayas
Coconut	Pears
Dates	Persimmons
Figs	Pineapple
Grapes	Plums

Meats and eggs

Whenever possible, choose meats and eggs from animals that were grass-fed and pasture-raised, and steer clear of meats that have been processed or cured with potentially toxic additives such as nitrites or nitrates.

Beef	Lamb
Chicken	Organ meats
Eggs (chicken, duck, quail, etc.)	Pork
Game meats (deer, elk, etc.)	Turkey
Goat	

Fish, shellfish, seafood

Any fish or shellfish is allowed on the Paleo diet, but you are advised to limit your consumption of high-mercury fish and, of course, to steer clear of fish or shellfish grown or obtained through ecologically unsustainable practices.

Anchovies	Crab
Arctic char	Lobster
Barramundi	Mackerel
Catfish	Mahimahi
Clams	Mussels
Cod	Oysters

Pollock

Salmon

Sea bass

Scallops

Shrimp/prawns

Snapper

Sole

Squid

Tilapia

Trout

Tuna

Nuts and seeds

While all nuts and seeds are on the "enjoy" list, as are butters or flours made from them (almond butter, cashew butter, almond flour, coconut flour, etc.), be aware that peanuts are not nuts, but legumes and they (and peanut butter) are on the "avoid" list. As with fruits, if you are trying to lose weight, nuts and seeds should be limited to just one or two small servings per day since they are high in calories.

Almonds

Cashews

Flaxseed

Hazelnuts

Macadamia nuts

Pecans

Sesame seeds

Sunflower seeds

Walnuts

Healthy fats

These fats are all Paleo-approved, but again, if you're trying to lose weight, consume them sparingly.

Avocado oil

Coconut oil/coconut milk/
    coconut butter

Grass-fed butter

Hazelnut oil

Lard (rendered pork fat)

Macadamia oil

Olive oil

Tallow (rendered beef fat)

Walnut oil

Enjoy only in moderation

Alcohol

Caffeinated tea

Chocolate (dark only)

Coffee

Dried fruit

Natural sweeteners (raw honey, stevia,
    coconut palm sugar, maple syrup)

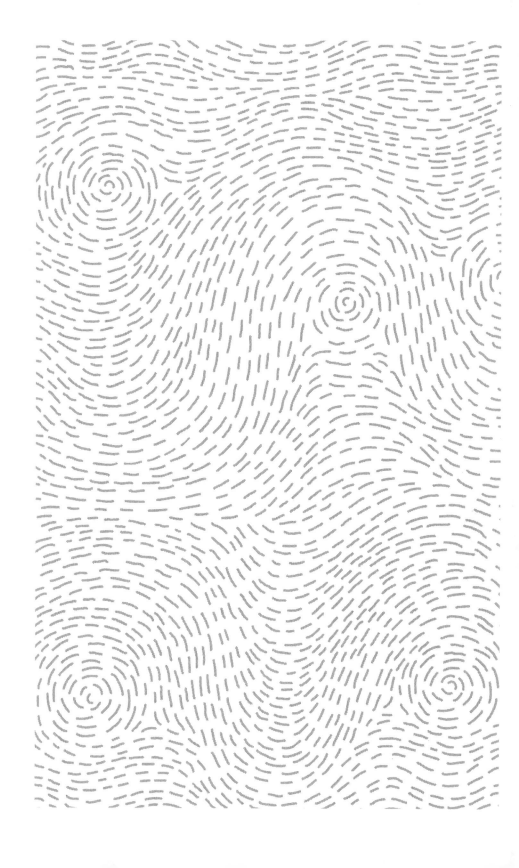

CHAPTER TWO

How to Save Time and Money

Now that you understand the theory behind the Paleo diet and how eating like an early human can greatly benefit your health and well-being, it's time to put the diet into action in your own life.

There are many sources of information—books, blogs, websites, etc.—about the Paleo diet. Many of these sources, unfortunately, assume that you have all the time in the world to research foods, seek out hard-to-find ingredients, and then pay through the nose for them, all in order to labor over complicated recipes. Rest assured, adopting the Paleo lifestyle does not require you to give up your day job or drain your savings account.

This chapter provides tips and advice for adopting a Paleo lifestyle—quickly, easily, and without breaking the bank. Here you'll find information on the handful of specialty ingredients that will prove good investments, plus advice on shopping for affordable Paleo-friendly ingredients. You'll learn about planning your meals, cooking, and stocking your pantry so that a delicious Paleo-friendly meal is always just minutes away.

PLAN AHEAD

As with any diet, meal plan, or lifestyle change, the key to success is planning ahead. To make the change to the Paleo way of eating, you'll need to stock up on certain Paleo-friendly foods and change up your day-to-day meal plan.

Start by planning out the meals you'll eat for the next week. Look through the recipes in this book, as well as those in other sources, and decide what you'll eat each day for breakfast, lunch, and dinner. Don't forget to think about snacks: both substantial snacks to serve as mini meals as needed throughout the day, as well as those little nibbles that tide you over between meals.

While it may seem time-consuming to write out a meal plan, it will ultimately save you time, not to mention money, to know exactly what you are going to eat and to get everything you need in one shopping trip.

When you are just starting out, be careful to write simple meal plans. Many of your meals can be put together out of basic ingredients, and leftovers can supply multiple meals. For instance, roast a chicken one night and serve it with roasted or steamed vegetables. The next day's breakfast can be scrambled eggs with leftover veggies. And for lunch, you can have a green salad with some of the chicken.

MAKE A SHOPPING LIST

Once you have your meal plan ready to go, make a detailed shopping list. Be sure to include every ingredient for every dish or snack you plan to prepare, checking your pantry as you go to see what you already have. You'll obviously want to include protein (meat, fish, shellfish), vegetables, fruits, nuts, and seeds.

As far as specialty ingredients, many Paleo cookbooks call for expensive oils, exotic nut flours and butters, and other pricey ingredients that may or may not be available at your local markets. The recipes in this book use mostly everyday ingredients that are available at your supermarket: meats, vegetables, fruits, nuts, seeds, honey, coconut or almond milk, herbs, and spices. Organic products are recommended whenever possible, and most supermarkets now carry these. A few of the more unusual ingredients that you'll likely want to invest in are coconut oil, coconut flour, coconut palm sugar, and almond flour.

Coconut oil is full of healthy fats and is one of the preferred cooking oils for Paleo dieters since it doesn't break down at high temperatures. Olive oil is okay to use for salad dressings and other non-cooked dishes, or in dishes that are not heated to high temperatures, but for high-temperature cooking, coconut oil is recommended. Look for unrefined, virgin, organic, cold-pressed coconut oil for the best quality. This can be found at natural food outlets, but many mainstream grocery stores carry it as well.

Coconut flour, coconut palm sugar, and almond flour make good substitutes for the conventional grain flours and refined sugars you find in many baking recipes. These items can be a bit pricey, but you usually use only a small amount for a dish (this is especially true of coconut flour), so a small package will last you a long while.

TIPS FOR ADOPTING THE PALEO DIET

Here are a few quick tips for preparing meals and snacks:

- Make sure your kitchen is equipped with good chopping knives, plus lidded containers and ziplock bags for holding the food items you prepare.
- Make sure you have skillets, sauté pans, and a soup pot for making your Paleo meals. You may want to invest in a slow cooker, which is a terrific tool for making several portions of Paleo-friendly dishes.
- Eat eggs for breakfast (and lunch and dinner, too!). Eggs are affordable, widely available, very nutritious, and easy to make. Scramble up a few with some healthy veggies for a quick breakfast, or make frittatas (see page 40), and keep them in your fridge or freezer for a grab-and-go breakfast on busy mornings. Hard-boil a bunch of eggs to have on hand in the fridge or your lunch bag for quick snacks.
- Salads are popular on the Paleo diet because they are satisfying, very nutritious, and can incorporate many different ingredients and flavors. Prep lots of salad vegetables and other ingredients at the beginning of the week so they are readily available all week long. Rinse and trim mixed greens, spinach, radishes, bell peppers, cucumbers, carrots, avocados, nuts, apples, pears, and meat or seafood. Store them in one large container or in individual containers so that you can make up a quick salad to take to work or for a fast lunch at home. Make salad dressing in a jar and store that in the fridge, too.
- Buy precut carrot and celery sticks, sliced fruit, and pre-portioned raw nut and/or dried fruit mixes for easy grab-and-go snacks. Or make your own portions, and keep them in the fridge or cupboard.
- Pre-prep fruits and veggies whenever possible. For instance, cut up a whole melon and store it in a sealed container in the fridge. When chopping an onion for a dish, go ahead and chop two or three onions, then store the extra in a ziplock bag in the fridge to use in other recipes that week.
- For dinner, certain meats and veggies are quick and easy to make, and offer endless variety. Try roasted, grilled, pan-seared, or braised meats, and raw, roasted, steamed, or grilled vegetables.
- If you really miss having a starchy or grain-based side dish, try substituting spaghetti squash or other vegetables (like zucchini "noodles") for pasta. You can also swap minced cauliflower for rice, or mashed cauliflower or winter squash for mashed potatoes.

- Plan your meals with leftovers in mind, so that one cooking session can feed you for several meals.
- Berries and other fruits make delicious, healthful desserts on their own. For a super special treat, top them with whipped coconut cream (see page 128).

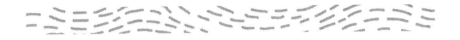

PART TWO

Quick and Easy Recipes

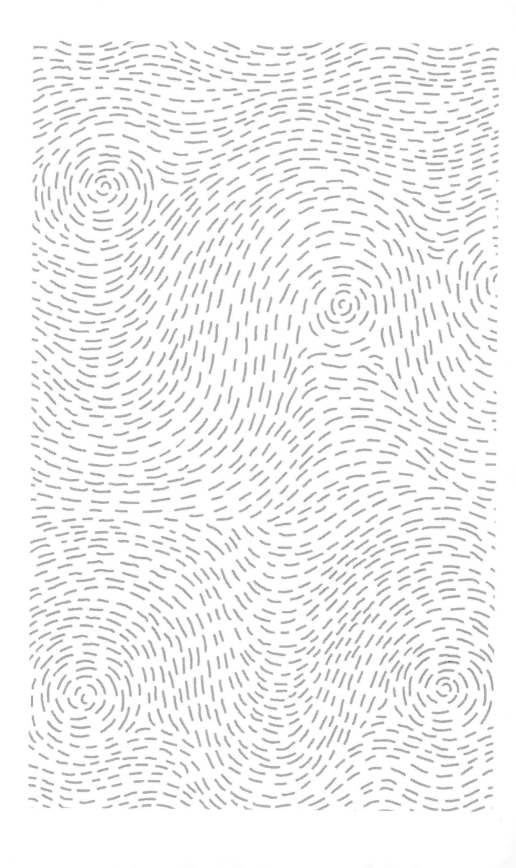

Breakfast

Very Berry Coconut Smoothie

Prep time: 5 minutes

Coconut yogurt is made from cultured coconut milk. It's dairy free, so it makes a great substitute for regular yogurt.

1½ CUPS FRESH OR FROZEN BERRIES, THAWED (BLUEBERRIES, STRAWBERRIES, BLACKBERRIES, RASPBERRIES, OR A COMBINATION)
½ CUP VANILLA COCONUT YOGURT
⅔ CUP COCONUT MILK
1 TABLESPOON GROUND FLAXSEED
1 TEASPOON HONEY

1. In a blender, combine all ingredients and process until smooth.

2. Serve immediately.

Banana-Chocolate Wake-Up Smoothie

SERVES 1

Prep time: 5 minutes

This quick shake is a delicious morning pick-me-up and the perfect accompaniment to an omelet or scrambled eggs. It also makes a good midmorning snack, providing sustenance and a kick of caffeine.

1 FROZEN BANANA, SLICED

½ CUP ICE CUBES

½ CUP STRONG BREWED COFFEE, AT ROOM TEMPERATURE OR FROZEN IN ICE CUBE TRAYS

2 TABLESPOONS COCOA POWDER

1 TABLESPOON HONEY

1 TABLESPOON COCONUT BUTTER

⅛ TEASPOON VANILLA EXTRACT (OPTIONAL)

1. In a blender, combine all ingredients and blend on high speed until smooth.

2. Serve immediately.

Grain-Free Granola Crunch

Prep time: 5 minutes
Cook time: 25 minutes

You won't miss the grains in this satisfying granola. Nuts and sunflower seeds give it crunch, while coconut offers chewy flakes.

COOKING SPRAY
1½ CUPS ALMOND FLOUR
½ CUP COCONUT OIL
¼ CUP HONEY
2 TEASPOONS GROUND CINNAMON
2 TEASPOONS VANILLA EXTRACT
¼ TEASPOON SALT
1 CUP SHREDDED COCONUT
1 CUP MIXED NUTS
¼ CUP SUNFLOWER SEEDS

1. Preheat the oven to 275°F. Coat a large baking sheet with cooking spray.

2. In a large bowl, combine the almond flour, coconut oil, honey, cinnamon, vanilla, salt, coconut, mixed nuts, and sunflower seeds, and mix well.

3. Spread the mixture in an even layer on the prepared baking sheet and bake, tossing once, until lightly browned and crisp, 20 to 25 minutes.

4. Let cool before serving. Store at room temperature in a sealed container for up to 1 week.

Grain-Free Hot Breakfast Cereal

SERVES 2

Prep time: 2 minutes
Cook time: 10 minutes

This simple cereal will fill the void left in your life when you gave up oatmeal. Top it with any number of delicious tidbits, like fresh berries, thawed frozen berries, toasted nuts, dried fruit, honey, maple syrup, cinnamon, or coconut milk.

1 RIPE BANANA, MASHED
3 EGGS
¼ CUP UNSWEETENED ALMOND OR COCONUT MILK
1 TEASPOON VANILLA EXTRACT
2 CUPS ALMOND FLOUR
1 TEASPOON GROUND CINNAMON

1. In a small saucepan over medium heat, warm the mashed banana.

2. While the banana is heating, in a small bowl, whisk the eggs, almond milk, and vanilla together. Add the egg mixture to the banana and stir to mix.

3. Slowly stir in the almond flour and cinnamon. Cover, reduce the heat to low, and let simmer, stirring occasionally, until thick and hot, about 5 minutes. Serve immediately.

Almond-Blueberry Muffins

Prep time: 5 minutes
Cook time: 25 minutes

Both almonds and blueberries are considered superfoods because of their high nutrient content. And they contain antioxidants, which are believed to strengthen the immune system and help prevent cancer. These muffins can be reheated in the microwave for a quick breakfast or snack.

2 CUPS ALMOND FLOUR

½ CUP TAPIOCA STARCH

½ TEASPOON BAKING SODA

½ TEASPOON BAKING POWDER

¼ TEASPOON SALT

⅓ CUP COCONUT SUGAR

¼ CUP GRASS-FED BUTTER, AT ROOM TEMPERATURE

2 TEASPOONS VANILLA EXTRACT

3 EGGS, AT ROOM TEMPERATURE

½ CUP PLAIN, UNSWEETENED ALMOND MILK

1½ CUPS FRESH BLUEBERRIES (OR 1 CUP FROZEN, THAWED)

¼ CUP SLICED ALMONDS, FOR GARNISH (OPTIONAL)

1. Preheat the oven to 350°F. Line a standard twelve-cup muffin tin with paper liners.

2. In a medium bowl, stir together the almond flour, tapioca starch, baking soda, baking powder, and salt. Set aside.

3. In a large bowl, using an electric mixer on medium speed, cream the coconut sugar and butter together until pale yellow and fluffy, about 5 minutes. Add the vanilla and eggs and beat another 1 or 2 minutes, until well combined.

4. Add the almond flour mixture to the egg mixture and beat to incorporate, about 1 minute. With the mixer running, slowly pour in the almond milk, beating until incorporated. Turn off the mixer. With a spoon, gently fold in the blueberries.

5. Spoon the batter into the prepared muffin tin, dividing it equally among the muffin cups. Sprinkle the sliced almonds over the top, if using. Bake until the tops begin to brown and a toothpick inserted into the center comes out clean, 20 to 25 minutes.

6. Cool on a wire rack and serve warm or at room temperature, or cool to room temperature and store in the refrigerator for up to 5 days, or in the freezer for up to 3 months.

Spiced Carrot Cake Muffins

Prep time: 5 minutes
Cook time: 25 minutes

Packed with beta-carotene-rich carrots and sweetened with just a touch of honey, these grain-free muffins are sure to please. Combining almond flour and coconut flour makes for just the right texture.

1½ CUPS BLANCHED ALMOND FLOUR

¾ CUP COCONUT FLOUR

2 TEASPOONS GROUND CINNAMON

¾ TEASPOON BAKING SODA

¼ TEASPOON GROUND GINGER

¼ TEASPOON SALT

⅛ TEASPOON GROUND NUTMEG

4 EGGS, AT ROOM TEMPERATURE

¾ CUP UNSWEETENED APPLESAUCE, AT ROOM TEMPERATURE

⅓ CUP HONEY

¼ CUP COCONUT OIL, MELTED

1 TEASPOON VANILLA EXTRACT

2 CUPS GRATED CARROTS

1. Preheat the oven to 350°F. Line a standard twelve-cup muffin tin with paper liners.

2. In a medium bowl, stir together the almond flour, coconut flour, cinnamon, baking soda, ginger, salt, and nutmeg. Set aside.

3. In a large bowl, combine the eggs, applesauce, honey, coconut oil, and vanilla. Whisk or stir to mix well.

4. Add the almond flour mixture to the egg mixture and stir just to combine. Stir in the carrots.

5. Spoon the batter into the prepared muffin tin, dividing it equally among the muffin cups. Bake until a toothpick inserted in the center comes out clean, 20 to 25 minutes.

6. Transfer the muffins to a wire rack to cool. Serve warm or at room temperature, or cool to room temperature and store in the refrigerator for up to 5 days, or in the freezer for up to 3 months.

Perfect Paleo Pancakes

Prep time: 5 minutes
Cook time: 15 minutes

These Paleo-friendly pancakes are free of grain, dairy, and refined sugars. Coconut flour may seem expensive, but it is drier and denser than wheat flour, so you need a lot less of it. A typical pancake recipe calls for about 1½ cups wheat flour, but this one requires only ½ cup of coconut flour. That 1-pound bag of coconut flour will last quite a while.

4 EGGS, AT ROOM TEMPERATURE

1 CUP COCONUT MILK, PLUS A BIT MORE FOR CONSISTENCY, IF NEEDED

2 TEASPOONS VANILLA EXTRACT

1 TABLESPOON HONEY

½ CUP COCONUT FLOUR, PLUS A BIT MORE FOR CONSISTENCY, IF NEEDED

1 TEASPOON BAKING SODA

½ TEASPOON SALT

¼ TEASPOON GROUND CINNAMON

2 TABLESPOONS COCONUT OIL

MAPLE SYRUP FOR SERVING, OR FRUIT (OPTIONAL)

1. In a large bowl, with an electric mixer, beat the eggs, coconut milk, vanilla, and honey until well mixed. Set aside.

2. In a small bowl, mix together the coconut flour, baking soda, salt, and cinnamon.

3. Add the flour mixture to the egg mixture and beat until well combined. If the mixture is too thick for pancakes, add a bit more coconut milk. If it is too runny, add a bit more coconut flour.

4. Heat a large skillet over medium-high heat and add the coconut oil. When the oil is hot, ladle the batter into the pan to make 3-inch pancakes. Cook until the underside is nicely browned, about 2 minutes. Flip over and cook until browned, another 2 minutes.

5. Serve hot, with maple syrup or fruit if desired.

Fluffy Almond-Banana Pancakes

SERVES 6

Prep time: 5 minutes
Cook time: 15 minutes

These simple, fluffy pancakes are every bit as delicious as their carb-heavy kin. Serve them topped with coconut yogurt, maple syrup, chopped nuts, or fresh fruit.

2 CUPS ALMOND FLOUR

3 RIPE BANANAS, MASHED

4 EGGS

½ CUP WATER

1 TEASPOON COCONUT OIL

1 TEASPOON HONEY

PINCH OF SALT

COOKING SPRAY

1. In a large bowl, combine the almond flour, bananas, eggs, water, oil, honey, and salt, and stir until well combined and smooth.

2. Coat a nonstick skillet with cooking spray and heat over medium-high heat.

3. Ladle the batter into the pan, about ¼ cup at a time. Cook until bubbles start to appear on top, about 2 minutes; then flip the pancakes over and cook until golden on the second side, about 2 minutes more. Repeat until all the batter has been cooked, adding cooking spray to the pan between batches as needed.

4. Serve immediately with desired toppings.

Crispy Cauliflower Fritters

Prep time: 10 minutes
Cook time: 15 minutes

Made of healthy veggies, nuts, seeds, and herbs, these crispy fritters are a Paleo dream. They are low in carbs and full of protein and fiber. You'll feel full and satisfied all morning long. Make extra, stash them in the fridge, and heat them in the microwave for a quick breakfast another day.

1 HEAD CAULIFLOWER, CORED AND CUT INTO SMALL FLORETS

2 CARROTS, GRATED

4 EGGS, LIGHTLY BEATEN

½ CUP FLAXSEED MEAL

½ CUP RAW, UNSALTED SUNFLOWER SEEDS

½ CUP HAZELNUTS, FINELY CHOPPED

½ CUP FRESH PARSLEY, FINELY CHOPPED

2 TEASPOONS FRESH LIME JUICE

1 TEASPOON SALT

½ TEASPOON WHITE PEPPER

2 TEASPOONS FRESH THYME

1 TEASPOON SMOKED PAPRIKA

½ TEASPOON CAYENNE PEPPER

2 TABLESPOONS COCONUT OIL, PLUS MORE FOR THE PAN IF NEEDED

1. Place the cauliflower in a food processor and pulse until it resembles coarse meal. Transfer to a large mixing bowl.

2. Add the carrots, eggs, flaxseed meal, sunflower seeds, hazelnuts, parsley, lime juice, salt, white pepper, thyme, paprika, and cayenne pepper, and mix well to combine.

continued ▶

3. Heat the oil in a medium nonstick skillet over medium-high heat. Ladle the batter into the pan about ¼ cup at a time. Flatten each round with the back of the ladle as it hits the pan.

4. Cook for about 3 minutes per side, until the fritters are golden brown. Repeat until you have used up all the batter, adding a bit more oil between batches if needed.

5. Serve immediately.

Avocado, Bacon, and Tomato Omelet

SERVES 2

Prep time: 5 minutes
Cook time: 10 minutes

Omelets are a great way to make simple ingredients into an elegant meal without a lot of fuss. In this dish, delicately cooked eggs are filled with smoky bacon, creamy avocado, and bright tomatoes.

1 TEASPOON COCONUT OIL

4 EGGS, BEATEN

1 TOMATO, DICED

½ AVOCADO, DICED

4 STRIPS BACON, COOKED AND CRUMBLED

¼ TEASPOON SALT

¼ TEASPOON PEPPER

2 TABLESPOONS CHOPPED CILANTRO, FOR GARNISH

1. Heat the oil in a medium nonstick skillet set over medium-high heat.

2. Add half of the eggs to the pan and cook until the edges begin to set. Using a spatula, push the set edges toward the center of the pan and tilt the pan to let the uncooked egg fill in around the outside.

3. When the eggs are nearly set, add half of the tomatoes, half of the avocado, and half of the bacon in a strip down the middle. Sprinkle ⅛ teaspoon of the salt and ⅛ teaspoon of the pepper on top.

4. Slide the omelet onto a plate, rolling half of the omelet over the other half.

5. Repeat steps 1–4 to make the second omelet. Serve immediately, garnished with cilantro.

Egg Muffins with Peppers, Onions, and Jalapeño

MAKES 12 MUFFINS

Prep time: 5 minutes
Cook time: 25 minutes

These tasty egg muffins are full of protein and healthy veggies. They are easy to make and they keep well in the fridge or freezer. Just pop them in a microwave to reheat.

1 TABLESPOON COCONUT OIL, PLUS MORE FOR THE MUFFIN TIN
1 YELLOW ONION, DICED
2 GARLIC CLOVES, MINCED
1 GREEN BELL PEPPER, DICED
1 RED BELL PEPPER, DICED
1 JALAPEÑO PEPPER, FINELY DICED
12 EGGS
1 TEASPOON SALT
½ TEASPOON PEPPER

1. Preheat the oven to 350°F. Brush a standard twelve-cup muffin pan with coconut oil.

2. Heat the tablespoon of coconut oil in a large skillet over medium-high heat. Add the onion and garlic and cook, stirring occasionally, until they soften, about 4 minutes. Add the green bell pepper, red bell pepper, and jalapeño pepper, and cook until softened, about another 3 minutes. Remove from the heat and let cool for a few minutes.

3. In a large bowl, whisk the eggs with the salt and pepper. Add the cooked vegetable mixture and stir to mix well.

4. Ladle the egg mixture into the prepared muffin tin, dividing it equally among the muffin cups. Bake until puffed and golden, 10 to 15 minutes. Serve hot, or cool to room temperature and store in the refrigerator for up to 5 days, or in the freezer for up to 3 months.

Eggs Baked in Mushroom-Prosciutto Bowls

SERVES 4

Prep time: 3 minutes
Cook time: 20 minutes

Prosciutto is a bit spendy, but it is well worth the price for its delicate texture and rich flavor. This recipe uses this elegant, thin ham to line egg-filled mushroom bowls. If you don't want to splurge on prosciutto, use thinly sliced ham instead.

4 PORTOBELLO MUSHROOM CAPS

1 TABLESPOON OLIVE OIL

4 SLICES OF PROSCIUTTO

4 EGGS

1 TEASPOON MINCED FRESH THYME

¼ TEASPOON SALT

¼ TEASPOON PEPPER

1. Preheat the oven to 350°F.

2. Remove the stems from the mushroom caps and scrape out the gills to make nice bowls. Brush the outside of each mushroom cap with olive oil and arrange them in a single layer, upside down, on a baking sheet.

3. Line the bowl of each mushroom cap with a slice of prosciutto, then crack an egg and drop it into each bowl. Sprinkle the tops with the thyme, salt, and pepper. Bake until the eggs are set and the mushrooms are soft, about 20 minutes. Serve hot.

Bacon-Crusted Mini Quiches with Mushrooms and Greens

Prep time: 5 minutes
Cook time: 25 minutes

These delicious breakfast quiches make a terrific on-the-go breakfast. They can be prepared in advance and stored in the fridge or freezer, then heated in the microwave just before you dash out the door.

8 STRIPS BACON

1 TABLESPOON COCONUT OIL, PLUS MORE FOR THE MUFFIN TIN

1 ONION, CHOPPED

3 OR 4 BUTTON OR CREMINI MUSHROOMS, CHOPPED

1 POUND SWISS CHARD, STEMMED AND CUT INTO RIBBONS

6 EGGS

¾ TEASPOON SALT

¼ TEASPOON PEPPER

1. Preheat the oven to 400°F. Lightly brush coconut oil on eight cups of a standard muffin tin.

2. Place a strip of bacon into each of the eight muffin cups, wrapping the bacon around the edge to form a bottomless cup. Set the muffin tin aside.

3. Heat the tablespoon of coconut oil in a medium skillet over medium-high heat. Add the onion and mushrooms and cook, stirring, until they begin to soften, about 3 minutes. Add the chard and cook until wilted, 3 to 4 minutes more. Remove from the heat and set aside.

4. In a large bowl, whisk the eggs with the salt and pepper until fluffy. Stir the vegetable mixture into the eggs until well combined; then ladle the mixture into the bacon-lined muffin cups, dividing it equally.

5. Bake until puffed and golden, about 20 minutes. Serve hot, or cool to room temperature and store in the refrigerator for up to 5 days, or in the freezer for up to 3 months.

Sweet Potato and Sausage Frittata

MAKES 8 SERVINGS

Prep time: 5 minutes
Cook time: 20 minutes

A frittata is a convenient way to cook up several meals' worth of eggs and pack them full of veggies. This one is also studded with bits of spicy sausage. Store extra servings in the fridge or freezer for breakfast on days when you have no time to cook.

3 TABLESPOONS COCONUT OIL

1 POUND ITALIAN SAUSAGE, GROUND OR REMOVED FROM CASINGS

1 SWEET POTATO, PEELED AND GRATED

4 GREEN ONIONS, THINLY SLICED

10 EGGS

¾ TEASPOON SALT

¼ TEASPOON PEPPER

1. Turn the oven on to broil. Put an oven rack about 5 inches below the broiler.

2. Heat the coconut oil in a large, oven-proof skillet over medium heat. Add the sausage and cook, stirring and breaking it up, until browned, about 5 minutes.

3. Add the sweet potato and continue to cook, stirring frequently, until softened, about 3 minutes. Stir in the green onions and cook until slightly softened, another 1 to 2 minutes.

4. Remove from the heat and distribute the mixture evenly across the skillet. Set aside.

5. Crack the eggs into a large bowl, add the salt and pepper, and whisk until frothy. Pour the eggs over the mixture in the skillet.

6. Over medium-high heat, cook the frittata until the edges are nearly set, about 3 minutes. Then transfer the skillet to the oven and broil until the eggs are lightly browned and completely set, 3 to 4 minutes.

7. Cut into wedges and serve hot. Or cool to room temperature, cut into wedges, wrap each wedge in plastic wrap, and store in the refrigerator for up to 5 days, or in the freezer for up to 3 months.

Quick Butternut Squash Hash

SERVES 4

Prep time: 10 minutes
Cook time: 20 minutes

Who needs toast when you've got a plate of this delicious and colorful—not to mention super nutritious—hash to nestle your eggs on?

1 TABLESPOON COCONUT OIL

2 GARLIC CLOVES, MINCED

2 CUPS DICED BUTTERNUT SQUASH

½ YELLOW ONION, DICED

SALT

PEPPER

1 RED, YELLOW, OR GREEN BELL PEPPER, DICED

1 TOMATO, FINELY CHOPPED

4 STRIPS NITRATE-FREE BACON, COOKED AND CRUMBLED

2 CUPS GENTLY PACKED FRESH SPINACH LEAVES

1. Heat the coconut oil in a large skillet over medium heat. Add the garlic and cook, stirring, for 1 minute.

2. Stir in the butternut squash, onion, and season with salt and pepper. Continue to cook, stirring frequently, for 5 minutes. Add the bell pepper and cook, stirring occasionally, for another 5 minutes. Add the tomato and bacon and cook, stirring occasionally, for 5 minutes more.

3. Stir in the spinach and cook until wilted, 2 to 3 minutes. Taste and adjust seasoning if needed. Serve immediately.

CHAPTER FOUR

Appetizers and Snacks

Kale Chips with a Kick

SERVES 4

Prep time: 5 minutes
Cook time: 15 minutes

Crispy, crunchy, and salty, these chips are a fantastic alternative to potato chips, or any salty snack you might be craving. Kale is one of the most nutrient-dense foods on the planet. These chips are a delicious way to help you meet your daily requirement of vegetables.

1 TEASPOON PAPRIKA
½ TEASPOON SALT
½ TEASPOON GROUND CORIANDER
½ TEASPOON GROUND CUMIN
¼ TEASPOON CAYENNE PEPPER
1 BUNCH CURLY-LEAF KALE
2 TABLESPOONS COCONUT OIL

1. Preheat the oven to 375°F.

2. In a small bowl, stir together the paprika, salt, coriander, cumin, and cayenne pepper. Set aside.

3. Make sure the kale is very dry. In a large bowl, tear the kale into bite-size pieces. Drizzle the coconut oil over the kale, and toss to coat.

4. Transfer the kale to a large rimmed baking sheet, and spread it in a single layer. Sprinkle the paprika mixture over the kale pieces.

5. Bake until crispy, 10 to 15 minutes. Serve immediately, or store in an airtight container at room temperature for up to 3 days.

Paleo Cauliflower "Popcorn"

SERVES 4

Prep time: 5 minutes
Cook time: 25 minutes

Corn is a grain, which makes popcorn a Paleo no-no. This cauliflower version is salty and crunchy and just as addictive as the traditional stuff. For real movie theater flavor, drizzle melted grass-fed butter over it before serving.

1 HEAD CAULIFLOWER, CUT INTO SMALL FLORETS
2 TABLESPOONS COCONUT OIL
1 TEASPOON SALT

1. Preheat the oven to 425°F. Line a large rimmed baking sheet with parchment paper.

2. In a large bowl, stir together the cauliflower, coconut oil, and salt, and toss to coat well.

3. Spread the cauliflower out in a single layer on the prepared baking sheet. Bake until golden brown and beginning to crisp, about 25 minutes. Serve immediately.

Crispy Baked Onion Rings

Prep time: 5 minutes
Cook time: 25 minutes

Batter-dipped, deep-fried, fast-food onion rings are addictive to be sure, but they go against just about every rule of Paleo eating. This simple oven-baked version is crispy, flavorful, and sure to keep people coming back for more. Better still, it is completely Paleo-friendly.

COCONUT OIL FOR THE BAKING SHEET
1 CUP COCONUT MILK
1 EGG
1 CUP ALMOND FLOUR
½ TEASPOON SALT, PLUS MORE IF NEEDED
¼ TEASPOON GARLIC POWDER
1 YELLOW ONION, CUT INTO ½-INCH-THICK SLICES AND SEPARATED
    INTO RINGS

1. Preheat the oven to 450°F. Lightly coat a large rimmed baking sheet with coconut oil.

2. In a medium shallow bowl, whisk together the coconut milk and egg. In a separate medium shallow bowl, stir together the almond flour, salt, and garlic powder.

3. Dip the onion rings, one at a time, first into the coconut milk mixture and then into the flour mixture. Arrange the battered onion rings on the prepared baking sheet in a single layer.

4. Bake for 15 minutes. Remove the pan from the oven and turn each onion ring over. Return to the oven and cook until golden brown and crispy, about 10 minutes.

5. Serve immediately, seasoned with additional salt, if desired.

Roasted Cauliflower Hummus

Prep time: 10 minutes
Cook time: 20 minutes

Traditional hummus made with chickpeas is off the Paleo menu, but this cauliflower version is just as delicious and satisfying. When roasted, cauliflower develops a deep, complex sweetness, and it blends into a velvety smooth purée.

2 TABLESPOONS COCONUT OIL

2 TEASPOONS GROUND CUMIN

1 TEASPOON PAPRIKA, PLUS MORE FOR GARNISH

½ TEASPOON SALT

1 HEAD CAULIFLOWER, CORED AND CUT INTO FLORETS

2 TABLESPOONS OLIVE OIL, PLUS MORE FOR GARNISH

½ CUP TAHINI

2 TABLESPOONS FRESH LEMON JUICE

4 GARLIC CLOVES, MINCED

1. Preheat the oven to 500°F. Line a large rimmed baking sheet with parchment paper.

2. In a large bowl, mix together the coconut oil, cumin, paprika, and salt. Add the cauliflower and toss to coat.

3. Spread the cauliflower out in a single layer on the prepared baking sheet. Roast until the cauliflower is soft and beginning to brown, about 20 minutes.

4. Transfer the cauliflower to a food processor. Add the 2 tablespoons of olive oil, tahini, lemon juice, and garlic and process to a smooth purée.

5. Serve the hummus topped with a drizzle of olive oil and a sprinkling of paprika.

Rosemary Crackers

MAKES ABOUT 24 CRACKERS

Prep time: 10 minutes
Cook time: 20 minutes

These crisp crackers are a great accompaniment to the Roasted Cauliflower Hummus (page 47) or the Cashew "Cheese" (page 49). You can change the flavor by using different herbs or spices: try thyme, oregano, cracked pepper, or garlic powder.

2 CUPS ALMOND FLOUR
½ TEASPOON SALT
2 TABLESPOONS MINCED FRESH ROSEMARY
1 EGG WHITE
2 TABLESPOONS WATER
1 TABLESPOON OLIVE OIL
¼ TEASPOON COCONUT OIL

1. Preheat the oven to 350°F.

2. In a medium bowl, stir together the almond flour, salt, and rosemary. Set aside.

3. In a separate medium bowl, whisk together the egg white, water, olive oil, and coconut oil.

4. Add the egg white mixture to the almond flour mixture, and stir well until a stiff dough forms.

5. Place a piece of parchment paper on your work surface and transfer the dough to it. Top with a second piece of parchment. With a rolling pin, roll the dough out to about ⅛ inch thick. Peel off the top piece of parchment paper, and transfer the bottom sheet, with the rolled dough on top, to a baking sheet. Trim the edges of the dough square using a pizza or pastry cutter; then cut the sheet of dough into 2-by-2-inch squares.

6. Bake for about 10 minutes. Turn off the oven, but leave the crackers inside to crisp up and turn golden brown for another 10 minutes. Transfer the crackers to a wire rack to cool. Serve at room temperature.

Cashew "Cheese"

Prep time: 5 minutes

For many, cheese is one of the hardest foods to give up. It's just such an easy snack and makes so many foods taste fantastic. This delicious dairy-free substitute will fill the void. Serve it with sliced apples, pears, or other fruits, or use it to top a Paleo-friendly pizza crust or plate of nachos.

1 CUP RAW CASHEWS, SOAKED IN WATER FOR AT LEAST 1 HOUR
　　AND DRAINED
¼ CUP WATER
1 TEASPOON FRESH LEMON JUICE
⅛ TEASPOON GARLIC POWDER
2 TABLESPOONS NUTRITIONAL YEAST FLAKES (OPTIONAL)
SALT
PEPPER

1. Place the drained cashews in a food processor and process until the nuts begin to break down.

2. Add the water, lemon juice, garlic powder, nutritional yeast (if using), and season with salt and pepper. Purée the mixture until it is very smooth. If the mixture is too thick, add a touch more water.

3. Serve immediately, or store, covered, in the refrigerator for up to 1 week.

Paleo Caprese Salad Bites

SERVES 4

Prep time: 5 minutes

Traditional caprese salad contains fresh mozzarella, which isn't Paleo-friendly. In this recipe, the cheese is replaced with rich, creamy avocado. These pretty little bites are like summer on a platter.

3 AVOCADOS, SLICED
JUICE OF 1 LEMON
4 HEIRLOOM TOMATOES, SLICED INTO ¼-INCH-THICK ROUNDS
SALT
PEPPER
1 BUNCH FRESH BASIL
OLIVE OIL

1. In a medium bowl, gently toss the avocado slices with the lemon juice.

2. Arrange the tomato slices in a single layer on a serving platter. Season lightly with salt.

3. Top each tomato slice with some slices of avocado, and season lightly with salt and pepper.

4. Top each tomato-avocado stack with a basil leaf and a drizzle of olive oil. Serve immediately.

Paleonnaise Salmon Salad–Stuffed Cucumber Canapés

MAKES ABOUT 16 CANAPÉS

Prep time: 15 minutes

Store-bought mayonnaise is full of Paleo-unfriendly ingredients—canola oil, corn oil, sugar, and preservatives, for starters. Paleonnaise is a delicious substitute that is a snap to make, especially if you have a stand mixer. Here it completes a spicy salmon salad that's stuffed into crisp cucumber rounds. This recipe makes more Paleonnaise than you need, so store the extra in a tightly sealed container in the fridge for up to 1 week and use it in tuna, egg, or chicken salads, deviled eggs, or anywhere you'd normally use mayonnaise. Feel free to substitute other Paleo-approved oils, such as avocado or macadamia, in the recipe.

PALEONNAISE

1 PASTEURIZED EGG YOLK

¼ TEASPOON SALT

¼ TEASPOON DIJON MUSTARD

1½ TEASPOONS FRESH LEMON JUICE

1 TEASPOON WHITE VINEGAR

¾ CUP OLIVE OIL

SALMON SALAD

¼ TEASPOON SMOKED PAPRIKA

¼ TEASPOON HOT PEPPER SAUCE

1 TABLESPOON CHOPPED CHIVES

SALT AND PEPPER

⅓ POUND COOKED SALMON, FLAKED

1 ENGLISH CUCUMBER, PEELED AND CUT CROSSWISE INTO ¾-INCH-THICK SLICES

4 CHERRY TOMATOES, QUARTERED

1 TABLESPOON CHOPPED FRESH CHIVES

continued ▶

For the Paleonnaise:

In a medium bowl, stand mixer, or blender, whisk together the egg yolk, salt, mustard, lemon juice, and vinegar. While whisking constantly, add the olive oil gradually in a very thin stream until the mixture is thick and emulsified, 3 to 4 minutes.

For the Salmon Salad:

1. In a medium bowl, combine ¼ cup of the Paleonnaise with the smoked paprika, hot pepper sauce, and chives. Season with salt and pepper and stir to mix well. Gently fold in the salmon.

2. Using a teaspoon or melon baller, scoop the seedy centers out of the cucumber slices, leaving a base on the bottom to form a cup. Arrange the cucumber cups on a serving platter. Spoon the salmon salad into the cucumber cups, dividing equally among the cups. Top each cup with a piece of tomato. Serve immediately, garnished with the chopped chives.

Smoky Prosciutto-Wrapped Squash Sticks

MAKES ABOUT 24 BITES

Prep time: 10 minutes
Cook time: 20 minutes

You often see recipes similar to this with shrimp in the middle. In this dish, butternut squash is a delicious and much more affordable stand-in. Prosciutto is a bit of a splurge, but you don't need a lot of it. If you want to trim costs even more, substitute bacon. You will need twenty-four wooden toothpicks that have been soaked in water for 10 minutes.

1 TABLESPOON COCONUT OIL

1 CLOVE GARLIC, MINCED

1 TEASPOON GROUND CHIPOTLE CHILE POWDER

1 TEASPOON BLACK PEPPER

¼ TEASPOON SALT

½ BUTTERNUT SQUASH, PEELED, SEEDED, AND CUT INTO FRENCH FRY-SHAPED STICKS

6 OUNCES VERY THINLY SLICED PROSCIUTTO, CUT INTO STRIPS

1. Preheat the oven to 350°F.

2. In a large bowl, stir together the coconut oil, garlic, chipotle, black pepper, and salt. Add the squash sticks and toss to coat well.

3. Wrap a squash stick with a strip of prosciutto. Secure with a toothpick and place on a baking sheet. Repeat with the remaining squash sticks and prosciutto.

4. Bake for approximately 20 minutes, turning once halfway through, until the prosciutto is crisp and the squash is tender. Serve immediately.

Chorizo-Stuffed Dates Wrapped in Bacon

MAKES 15 STUFFED DATES

Prep time: 10 minutes
Cook time: 15 minutes

Dates are naturally sweet and full of rich flavor that pairs nicely with both smoky bacon and spicy chorizo. The maple glaze in this recipe adds that extra touch that turns a simple dish into an elegant—and addictive—party-worthy appetizer. Secure the dates with toothpicks that have been soaked in water for 10 minutes.

15 PITTED MEDJOOL DATES
1 POUND SPANISH-STYLE CHORIZO, CUT INTO 15 PIECES
5 SLICES BACON, CUT INTO THIRDS
½ CUP MAPLE SYRUP

1. Preheat the oven to 400°F. Line a rimmed baking sheet with parchment paper.

2. Stuff a piece of chorizo inside each date (if necessary, make an incision on one side). Press the date together at the opening to close. Wrap each date with a bacon piece and stick a toothpick through it to secure.

3. Place the dates on the prepared baking sheet and roast until the bacon begins to get crispy, 5 to 6 minutes. Turn the dates over and cook until the bacon begins to crisp on the second side, about 6 more minutes.

4. Pour the maple syrup into a small, shallow bowl. Remove the dates from the oven (leave the oven on) and, holding onto the toothpick, dip each date into the bowl of maple syrup, coating it evenly on all sides. Return the dates to the pan.

5. Place the pan back in the oven and cook until the maple syrup has turned into a sticky glaze, about 2 minutes. Serve immediately.

Crispy Pepperoni Pizza Bites

SERVES 8 (MAKES ABOUT 24 MINI PIZZAS)

Prep time: 10 minutes
Cook time: 20 minutes

Who needs pizza crust when you've got crispy rounds of spicy pepperoni? Use a preservative-free pepperoni and dairy-free sun-dried tomato pesto (or just chopped sun-dried tomatoes packed in oil) to keep it Paleo. For a milder version, substitute salami for the pepperoni. If you've got leftover Cashew "Cheese" (see page 49), add a dollop on top before reheating.

6 OUNCES LARGE, SLICED PEPPERONI
½ CUP SUN-DRIED TOMATO PESTO OR MINCED OIL-PACKED (DRAINED) SUN-DRIED TOMATOES
½ CUP FINELY DICED MUSHROOMS
½ CUP CHOPPED FRESH BASIL

1. Preheat the oven to 400°F.

2. Arrange the slices of pepperoni in a single layer on a rimmed baking sheet. Bake for about 8 minutes until crispy, turning the slices over halfway through.

3. Remove from the oven (leave the oven on) and top each pepperoni slice with about 1 teaspoon of the sun-dried tomato pesto or diced sun-dried tomatoes. Sprinkle about 1 teaspoon of the mushrooms over the top.

4. Return to the oven and bake for another 5 to 10 minutes, until the pesto is hot and bubbly and the mushrooms are cooked.

5. Serve immediately, garnished with the basil.

Cocktail Meatballs

Prep time: 10 minutes
Cook time: 20 minutes

These sweet and sour meatballs are grain-free, and sweetened only with pineapple and pineapple juice. They're sure to be a hit at your next cocktail party.

1⅓ POUNDS GROUND TURKEY

3 GARLIC CLOVES, MINCED

1 TABLESPOON MINCED, PEELED FRESH GINGER

SALT

PEPPER

1 TABLESPOON COCONUT OIL

1 RED BELL PEPPER, CUT INTO 1-INCH SQUARES

ONE 20-OUNCE CAN PINEAPPLE CHUNKS IN JUICE

1 TABLESPOON ARROWROOT POWDER

1 BUNCH GREEN ONIONS, GREEN AND WHITE PARTS THINLY SLICED

1. Preheat the oven to 400°F.

2. In a medium bowl, combine the ground turkey, garlic, and ginger; season with salt and pepper, and mix well. Form the mixture into about thirty-six 1-inch meatballs and arrange them on a rimmed baking sheet. Bake the meatballs for about 15 minutes.

3. While the meatballs are baking, in a large skillet over medium-high heat, heat the coconut oil. Add the bell pepper and cook, stirring frequently, until softened, about 4 minutes. Add the pineapple, along with the juice, and cook until the pineapple is hot and the liquid is slightly reduced, about 5 minutes more.

4. In a small bowl, stir the arrowroot with a bit of water to make a slurry. Add the arrowroot slurry to the bell pepper–pineapple mixture, remove from heat, and stir until the sauce thickens.

5. When the meatballs are finished baking, add them to the skillet and toss to coat. Turn the meatballs and their sauce out onto a serving dish, garnish with the green onions, and serve with toothpicks.

Paleo Power Balls

Prep time: 10 minutes

These sweet little balls are just what you need to get you through a long after-noon. Medjool dates are especially moist and sweet, which is why they are recommended here. You can use other types of dates, but you may need to add a bit of honey for moisture and sweetness.

1¼ CUPS RAW WHOLE ALMONDS
1 POUND PITTED MEDJOOL DATES, COARSELY CHOPPED
1 TABLESPOON WATER
1½ TEASPOONS VANILLA
1 TEASPOON GROUND CINNAMON
1 TEASPOON ORANGE ZEST
¾ TEASPOON SALT
VEGETABLE OIL, FOR YOUR HANDS

1. Preheat the oven to 350°F.

2. Spread the almonds in a single layer on a large rimmed baking sheet, and toast them in the oven until they just begin to brown and become fragrant, about 5 minutes.

3. Place the almonds in a food processor, and pulse until finely ground. Transfer half of the ground almonds to a small shallow bowl and set aside.

4. Add the dates to the ground almonds in the food processor, along with the water, vanilla, cinnamon, orange zest, and salt. Process until the dates are very finely chopped and all of the ingredients are well mixed.

5. Coat your hands with a bit of vegetable oil and shape the mixture into 1½-inch balls. Roll the balls in the reserved ground almonds. Serve immediately, or store in plastic wrap in the refrigerator for up to 1 week.

Almond-Chai Bites

MAKES 24 BITES

Prep time: 30 minutes (includes chilling time)

Full of healthful nuts and seeds, these yummy snack bites will give you lots of energy. Feel free to substitute different nuts, nut butters, or dried fruits if you're feeling creative.

COCONUT OIL OR COCONUT OIL SPRAY FOR GREASING PAN

1 CUP RAW ALMONDS

1 CUP RAW SUNFLOWER SEEDS

2 TEASPOONS GROUND CINNAMON

1 TEASPOON GROUND GINGER

½ TEASPOON GROUND CARDAMOM

½ TEASPOON SALT

1 CUP UNSWEETENED SHREDDED COCONUT

½ CUP RAISINS

¼ CUP CREAMY RAW ALMOND BUTTER

¼ CUP HONEY

¼ CUP UNSWEETENED APPLESAUCE

2 TABLESPOONS GROUND FLAXSEED

1. Coat a mini muffin tin with coconut oil.

2. In the bowl of a food processor, combine the almonds, sunflower seeds, cinnamon, ginger, cardamom, and salt, and pulse several times until the nuts are finely chopped. Transfer to a large bowl, add the coconut and raisins, and stir to mix well. Set aside.

3. In a small saucepan over medium heat, combine the almond butter, honey, and applesauce, and whisk constantly, until the almond butter has melted and the mixture is smooth.

continued ▶

Almond-Chai Bites *continued* ▶

4. Stir in the flaxseed and pour the mixture over the nut mixture in the bowl. Stir to mix well.

5. Wet your hands slightly and press the mixture into the prepared mini muffin tin, dividing the mixture evenly among the muffin cups, pressing firmly to tightly pack each cup. Place the muffin tin in the freezer for about 20 minutes, until the bites are firm.

6. Serve immediately, or transfer to an airtight container and refrigerate for up to 1 week, or freeze for up to 3 months.

Quick Maple-Cinnamon Pecan Brittle

SERVES 6

Prep time: 5 minutes
Cook time: 20 minutes

These sweet-savory nut bites make a tasty snack or cocktail nibble. They also add a nice crunch to salads or, wrapped up with a pretty bow, make a lovely homemade gift. You can substitute other nuts, such as walnuts, to the recipe.

1 EGG WHITE

¼ CUP MAPLE SYRUP

1 TEASPOON SALT

1 TEASPOON GROUND CINNAMON

2 CUPS PECAN HALVES

1. Preheat the oven to 350°F. Line a large rimmed baking sheet with parchment paper.

2. In a large bowl, whisk together the egg white, maple syrup, salt, and cinnamon. Add the pecan halves, and toss to coat.

3. Transfer the pecan mixture to the prepared baking sheet, and spread it out in a single layer.

4. Bake until the nuts are nicely browned, about 20 minutes. Remove from the oven and let cool for 5 minutes.

5. Break the brittle into pieces and serve immediately, or store in an airtight container on the countertop for up to 1 week.

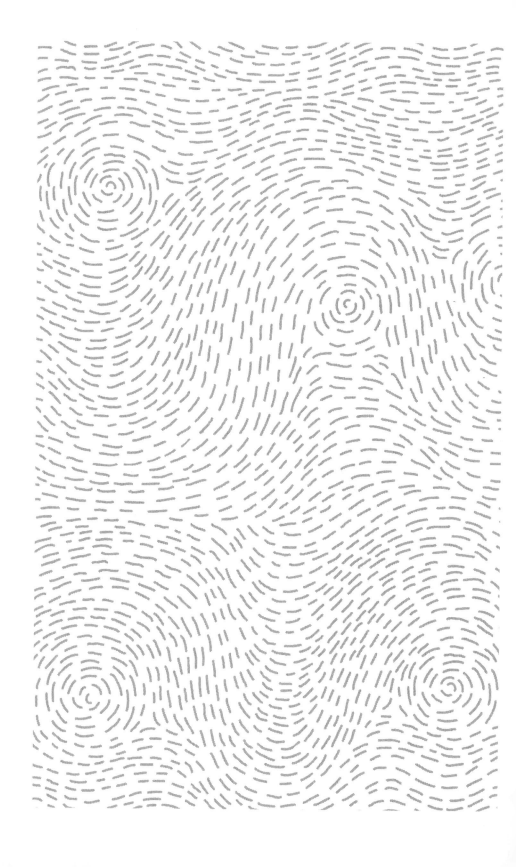

CHAPTER FIVE

Soups and Salads

Butternut Squash and Apple Soup

SERVES 6

Prep time: 5 minutes
Cook time: 25 minutes

Butternut squash is full of dietary fiber, as well as potassium, vitamin B6, and folate. It is also delicious and makes a beautifully orange-hued soup that, along with apples, makes a festive fall dish.

2 TABLESPOONS COCONUT OIL

1 ONION, DICED

1 BUTTERNUT SQUASH, PEELED, SEEDED, AND CUBED (ABOUT 6 CUPS)

ONE 16-OUNCE CAN COCONUT MILK

2 CUPS APPLE CIDER

2 APPLES, PEELED, CORED, AND CUBED

1 CARROT, CHOPPED

1 TEASPOON SALT

1 TEASPOON GROUND CINNAMON

½ TEASPOON GROUND NUTMEG

2 TABLESPOONS MINCED FRESH CHIVES

1. In a large stockpot over medium-high heat, heat the coconut oil. Add the onion and cook, stirring, until softened, about 5 minutes.

2. Add the squash, coconut milk, cider, apples, carrot, salt, cinnamon, and nutmeg, and bring to a boil. Reduce the heat to low, cover, and let simmer until the apples and squash are tender, about 20 minutes.

3. Purée the soup using an immersion blender or in batches in a countertop blender.

4. Return the soup to the pot, if necessary, and cook, stirring occasionally, over medium heat, until thoroughly heated through. Serve immediately, garnished with the chives.

Cream of Artichoke and Spinach Soup

Prep time: 5 minutes
Cook time: 20 minutes

Coconut cream stands in for the dairy you'd normally use to make this soup creamy. Asian markets often sell cans of coconut cream, but if you can't find it, simply chill a regular can of full-fat coconut milk (overnight if you've got time), open it, and scoop off the thick cream that has risen to the top (discarding the coconut water or saving it for another use). You'll get about 1 cup of cream from a 16-ounce can of coconut milk.

2 TABLESPOONS COCONUT OIL

1 ONION, CHOPPED

2 GARLIC CLOVES, COARSELY CHOPPED

10 OUNCES FRESH BABY SPINACH (ABOUT 6 GENTLY PACKED CUPS)

ONE 14-OUNCE CAN ARTICHOKE HEARTS, DRAINED

3 CUPS CHICKEN OR VEGETABLE BROTH

1 TEASPOON SALT

½ TEASPOON PEPPER

1 CUP COCONUT CREAM

1. In a large stockpot over medium-high heat, heat the coconut oil. Add the onion and cook, stirring frequently, until softened, about 5 minutes. Add the garlic and continue to cook, stirring, for 1 minute more. Stir in the spinach and artichoke hearts and cook until the spinach wilts, about 2 minutes.

2. Add the broth, salt, and pepper and bring to a boil. Reduce the heat to low and simmer, uncovered, for 10 minutes.

3. Stir the coconut cream into the soup.

4. Purée the soup with an immersion blender or in batches in a countertop blender.

5. Return the soup to the pot if necessary and reheat. Serve hot.

Leek, Fennel, and Turnip Soup

Prep time: 5 minutes
Cook time: 25 minutes

Turnips thicken this soup instead of the usual potatoes and cream. As a result, the soup is lighter but no less satisfying. The fennel gives the soup a rich and distinctive flavor.

2 TABLESPOONS COCONUT OIL

3 LEEKS, CLEANED AND THINLY SLICED

4 STALKS CELERY, THINLY SLICED

3 WHITE ONIONS, PEELED AND HALVED

1 BULB FENNEL, CORED AND THINLY SLICED

2 TURNIPS, PEELED AND CUT INTO ½-INCH CUBES

1 TABLESPOON SALT

1½ TEASPOONS PEPPER

8 CUPS VEGETABLE OR CHICKEN BROTH

1. In a large stockpot over medium heat, heat the coconut oil. Add the leeks, celery, onions, fennel, turnips, salt, and pepper, and cook, stirring frequently, for about 5 minutes, until the vegetables begin to soften.

2. Add the broth and bring to a boil. Reduce the heat to low and simmer, uncovered, until the vegetables are tender and the soup has begun to thicken, about 20 minutes.

3. Purée the soup using an immersion blender or in batches in a countertop blender. Return the soup to the pot if necessary and reheat.

4. Serve hot.

Mexican Chicken Soup

Prep time: 10 minutes
Cook time: 20 minutes

This simple soup is based on the classic chicken tortilla soup that is made with tortillas and, usually, beans. This version has no grains or legumes, but still offers plenty of spicy Mexican flavor.

2 TABLESPOONS COCONUT OIL

1 ONION, DICED

4 GARLIC CLOVES, MINCED

2 JALAPEÑO PEPPERS, DICED

2 POBLANO CHILES, DICED

1 TEASPOON GROUND CUMIN

1 TEASPOON MILD CHILI POWDER

1 TEASPOON DRIED OREGANO

1 TEASPOON SALT

½ TEASPOON BLACK PEPPER

¼ TEASPOON CAYENNE PEPPER

8 CUPS CHICKEN BROTH

ONE 28-OUNCE CAN DICED TOMATOES, DRAINED

2 POUNDS COOKED, SHREDDED CHICKEN BREAST MEAT

JUICE OF 2 LIMES

1 CUP CHOPPED FRESH CILANTRO, PLUS MORE FOR GARNISH

½ AVOCADO, DICED, FOR GARNISH

1. In a large stockpot over medium-high heat, heat the coconut oil. Add the onion and cook, stirring frequently, until soft, about 5 minutes.

continued ▶

2. Add the garlic, jalapeños, and poblanos, and cook, stirring frequently, for about 2 minutes. Stir in the cumin, chili powder, oregano, salt, black pepper, and cayenne pepper. Add the broth and tomatoes and bring to a boil.

3. Add the chicken and cook until heated through, about 10 minutes. Just before serving, stir in the lime juice and cilantro.

4. Serve hot, garnished with cilantro and diced avocado.

Tom Ka Gai (Thai Chicken–Coconut Milk Soup)

SERVES 6

Prep time: 10 minutes
Cook time: 20 minutes

Many Thai foods are easily adapted to suit a Paleo diet since they don't include dairy and, unlike dishes from many other Asian cuisines, they rarely include soy products. The common Thai grains, usually rice or rice noodles, are easily left out. This quick soup is very flavorful and offers a good dose of healthy fats from the coconut oil and coconut milk.

1 TABLESPOON COCONUT OIL

3 SHALLOTS, CHOPPED

2 TEASPOONS THAI RED CURRY PASTE

TWO 14-OUNCE CANS COCONUT MILK

4 CUPS CHICKEN BROTH

1 TABLESPOON HONEY

8 SPRIGS FRESH CILANTRO, CHOPPED

1 HEAD BROCCOLI, CUT INTO SMALL FLORETS

½ POUND BUTTON OR CREMINI MUSHROOMS

2 SKINLESS, BONELESS CHICKEN BREASTS HALVED LENGTHWISE AND
    SLICED AGAINST THE GRAIN INTO 1/8-INCH-THICK STRIPS

3 TABLESPOONS FRESH LIME JUICE

3 TABLESPOONS FISH SAUCE

½ CUP MINCED FRESH CILANTRO, FOR GARNISH

2 SERRANO CHILES, THINLY SLICED, FOR GARNISH

1 LIME, CUT INTO WEDGES, FOR GARNISH

continued ▶

Tom Ka Gai (Thai Chicken–Coconut Milk Soup) *continued* ▶

1. In a large stockpot over medium heat, heat the coconut oil. Add the shallots and cook, stirring frequently, until softened, about 5 minutes. Stir in the curry paste and cook, stirring, 1 minute more.

2. Add the coconut milk, broth, honey, and cilantro and bring to a boil. Reduce the heat to low and simmer for about 5 minutes.

3. Strain the broth through a fine mesh sieve, discard the solids, and return the broth to the stockpot over medium heat.

4. Add the mushrooms and broccoli, and cook until they begin to soften, about 5 minutes. Add the chicken, and cook until fully opaque and cooked through, about 5 minutes more.

5. Just before serving, add the lime juice and fish sauce. Serve hot, garnished with the minced cilantro, chile slices, and lime wedges.

Tuscan Sausage and Greens Soup

SERVES 6

Prep time: 5 minutes
Cook time: 25 minutes

Turnips and almond milk stand in for the Paleo-prohibited potatoes and cream normally found in this soup—making it every bit as delicious as the original.

1 POUND ITALIAN GROUND SAUSAGE, OR SAUSAGE WITHOUT
  THE CASINGS
1 ONION, DICED
3 GARLIC CLOVES, DICED
1 TEASPOON CRUSHED RED PEPPER FLAKES (OPTIONAL)
8 CUPS CHICKEN BROTH
4 TURNIPS, PEELED AND DICED
4 CUPS CHOPPED KALE, STEMS AND TOUGH CENTER RIBS REMOVED
ONE 32-OUNCE BOX UNSWEETENED ALMOND MILK
1 TEASPOON SALT
½ TEASPOON BLACK PEPPER

1. In a large stockpot over medium-high heat, cook the sausage, stirring to break up the meat, until thoroughly browned, about 5 minutes.

2. Add the onion and garlic and cook, stirring frequently, until softened, about 5 minutes. Stir in the red pepper flakes, if using.

3. Add the broth and turnips and bring to a boil. Reduce the heat to low and simmer, uncovered, for about 10 minutes. Stir in the kale and almond milk and continue to simmer until the turnips and kale are tender, and the soup is heated through, about 5 minutes more.

4. Season with salt and pepper and serve hot.

Classic Beef and Vegetable Soup

SERVES 4

Prep time: 5 minutes
Cook time: 25 minutes

This hearty classic soup will satisfy any appetite. It's quick and easy to make, and full of nutritious veggies and protein-rich beef.

2 POUNDS LEAN GROUND BEEF

1 ONION, DICED

3 CARROTS, SLICED INTO ½-INCH ROUNDS

2 CELERY STALKS, SLICED INTO ½-INCH PIECES

6 GARLIC CLOVES, MINCED

3 CUPS CHOPPED CABBAGE

ONE 15-OUNCE CAN DICED TOMATOES WITH THEIR JUICE

4 CUPS BEEF BROTH

1 TABLESPOON MINCED FRESH THYME

2 BAY LEAVES

½ TEASPOON SALT, PLUS MORE IF NEEDED

½ TEASPOON PEPPER, PLUS MORE IF NEEDED

¼ CUP CHOPPED FRESH FLAT-LEAF ITALIAN PARSLEY, FOR GARNISH

1. In a large stockpot over medium-high heat, cook the beef, stirring and breaking up the meat, until thoroughly browned, about 5 minutes.

2. Add the onion, carrots, celery, and garlic, and cook, stirring frequently, until the vegetables begin to soften, about 5 minutes. Add the cabbage, tomatoes along with their juice, and broth, and bring to a boil.

3. Stir in the thyme, bay leaves, salt, and pepper, cover, and reduce the heat to low.

4. Simmer for about 15 minutes. Taste and adjust seasoning as needed. Remove bay leaves and serve hot, garnished with the parsley.

Broccoli Crunch Salad with Warm Bacon Vinaigrette

SERVES 4

Prep time: 10 minutes
Cook time: 10 minutes

Broccoli—with its high vitamin and fiber content—is reported to help lower blood pressure and reduce the risk of heart disease and cancer. Paired with crisp apples, crunchy nuts, and smoky bacon in a warm vinaigrette, it is tasty and satisfying.

2 HEADS OF BROCCOLI, CUT INTO SMALL FLORETS (4 TO 5 CUPS)
½ RED ONION, THINLY SLICED
2 CRISP APPLES, THINLY SLICED
8 SLICES OF BACON
1 SHALLOT, FINELY DICED
1 TEASPOON DIJON MUSTARD
1 TABLESPOON APPLE CIDER VINEGAR
½ TEASPOON SALT
½ TEASPOON PEPPER
2 TABLESPOONS CHOPPED PECANS OR WALNUTS

1. Bring a large pot of salted water to a boil. Add the broccoli florets and cook for about 1 minute, just long enough to blanch. Drain and transfer immediately to a bowl of ice water to stop the cooking. Drain again and place in a large salad bowl. Add the onion and apples, mix to combine, and set aside.

2. In a large skillet over medium-high heat, cook the bacon, turning once or twice, until crisp, about 5 minutes. Transfer the bacon to a paper towel–lined plate to drain, and crumble when cool enough to handle. Retain about 3 tablespoons of the bacon fat in the skillet and discard the rest.

continued ▶

3. Turn the heat down to medium. Add the shallot to the hot bacon fat in the skillet and cook until it begins to soften, about 3 minutes. Remove skillet from the heat and immediately whisk in the mustard, vinegar, salt, and pepper until well combined.

4. Pour the warm bacon fat dressing over the broccoli-apple-onion mixture and toss well to coat. Add the crumbled bacon and chopped nuts and toss again. Serve immediately, while still warm.

Mexican Chicken Salad with Chipotle-Avocado Dressing

SERVES 4

Prep time: 15 minutes

Using avocado is a great way to make a creamy, rich salad dressing without dairy products. It offers healthy fats and other nutrients, tastes delicious, and makes a stunning green dressing for a fresh salad. Crisp jicama and radishes add a satisfying crunch, so you won't miss the crispy tortilla chips.

DRESSING

1 GARLIC CLOVE

1 AVOCADO

¼ CUP WATER

3 TABLESPOONS FRESHLY SQUEEZED LIME JUICE (FROM ABOUT 2 LIMES)

3 TABLESPOONS OLIVE OIL

¼ TEASPOON GROUND CHIPOTLE POWDER

1 TEASPOON SALT

SALAD

1 HEAD ROMAINE LETTUCE, TORN INTO BITE-SIZE PIECES

6 RADISHES, TRIMMED AND THINLY SLICED

1 RED BELL PEPPER, DICED

1 JICAMA, PEELED AND DICED

½ RED ONION, DICED

¾ POUND COOKED SKINLESS CHICKEN BREAST, SHREDDED OR CUT INTO BITE-SIZE PIECES

continued ▶

For the Dressing:

Mince the garlic in a food processor or blender. Halve the avocado and scoop the flesh into the food processor. Add the water, lime juice, olive oil, chipotle, and salt, and process to a smooth, pourable purée. If the dressing is too thick, add a bit more water or lime juice. Set aside.

For the Salad:

1. In a large salad bowl, toss together the lettuce, radishes, bell pepper, jicama, and red onion. Add the chicken and toss again to combine.

2. Pour the dressing over the salad and toss to coat. Serve immediately.

Cobb Salad

Prep time: 15 minutes

This Cobb salad is loaded with protein—from chicken, bacon, hard-boiled eggs, and pecans—making it a wonderful meal-size salad. Fortunately, it also has lots of nutritious veggies, fiber, and healthy fats. Blue cheese is the mark of a Cobb salad, but to keep it strictly Paleo, this version substitutes diced apples and chopped pecans.

DRESSING

⅓ CUP OLIVE OIL

¼ CUP RED WINE VINEGAR

1 SHALLOT, MINCED

1 TABLESPOON FRESH LEMON JUICE

2 TEASPOONS DIJON MUSTARD

¾ TEASPOON SALT

½ TEASPOON PEPPER

SALAD

1 HEAD ROMAINE LETTUCE, CHOPPED

8 OUNCES COOKED CHICKEN BREAST, DICED OR SHREDDED

2 EGGS, HARD-BOILED, PEELED, AND CHOPPED

2 TOMATOES, DICED

1 CUCUMBER, PEELED, SEEDED, AND SLICED

1 CRISP APPLE, DICED

½ AVOCADO, DICED

2 TABLESPOONS CHOPPED PECANS

2 SLICES COOKED BACON, CRUMBLED

continued ▶

Cobb Salad *continued* ▶

For the Dressing:

In a small bowl, whisk together the olive oil, vinegar, shallot, lemon juice, mustard, salt, and pepper until well combined. Set aside.

For the Salad:

1. Place the romaine in a large mixing bowl. Drizzle with half of the dressing and toss to coat. Arrange the lettuce on four serving plates. Arranging each ingredient in a line, top the romaine with the chicken, eggs, tomatoes, cucumber, apple, avocado, pecans, and bacon.

2. Drizzle the remaining dressing over the salads and serve immediately.

Composed Lox and Egg Salad

SERVES 4

Prep time: 15 minutes

Bagels and cream cheese may be off the menu, but that doesn't mean you have to give up lox. This flavorful salad is perfect for a Sunday brunch or a light lunch any day of the week.

DRESSING

2 TABLESPOONS FRESH LEMON JUICE

½ TEASPOON DIJON MUSTARD

½ TEASPOON KOSHER SALT

¼ CUP OLIVE OIL

SALAD

4 OUNCES LOX, CUT INTO STRIPS

4 HARD-BOILED EGGS, PEELED AND CHOPPED

1 AVOCADO, DICED

½ ENGLISH CUCUMBER, THINLY SLICED

10 CHERRY TOMATOES, HALVED OR QUARTERED

¼ RED ONION, THINLY SLICED

2 TABLESPOONS CAPERS, DRAINED

FRESHLY GROUND PEPPER, TO SERVE

For the Dressing:

Combine the lemon juice, mustard, and salt in a small bowl and whisk to combine. Whisk in the olive oil until the dressing is well combined and emulsified. Set aside.

For the Salad:

1. On a serving platter or on individual salad plates, arrange the lox, eggs, avocado, cucumber, tomatoes, and red onion. Top with the capers and a generous dose of freshly ground pepper.

2. Drizzle the dressing over the salad. Serve immediately.

Grilled Romaine and Bacon Salad

SERVES 4

Prep time: 5 minutes
Cook time: 20 minutes

Most Paleo eaters consume a lot of salads. Grilling the lettuce offers an interesting twist. Topping the grilled lettuce with garlicky tomatoes and crisp bacon take this salad over the top.

2 TEASPOONS OLIVE OIL

2 HEADS ROMAINE LETTUCE, HALVED LENGTHWISE

8 STRIPS BACON

2 TOMATOES, DICED

2 GARLIC CLOVES, MINCED

2 TABLESPOONS CHOPPED FRESH FLAT-LEAF PARSLEY, FOR GARNISH

½ LEMON, FOR GARNISH

1. Heat a grill pan over medium-high heat and brush the olive oil on the grill pan.

2. Place the romaine halves, cut-side down, on the grill pan. Place an oven-proof heavy plate or pan lid on top of the romaine to ensure that the lettuce is making full contact with the grill. Cook until the lettuce is charred, about 10 minutes.

3. While the lettuce is grilling, heat a medium skillet over medium-high heat, and cook the bacon until crispy, about 4 minutes. Transfer the bacon to paper towels to drain, and when cool enough to handle, crumble the bacon.

4. Add the tomatoes to the bacon grease in the skillet and cook until they begin to break down, about 4 minutes. Add the garlic and cook, stirring frequently, until softened, 3 or 4 minutes.

5. To serve, place a grilled lettuce wedge on each of four serving plates. Top with the tomato mixture, dividing equally, and then sprinkle the bacon over the top.

6. Serve immediately, garnished with the parsley and a squeeze of lemon juice.

Cauliflower "Rice" Salad with Lemon-Herb Vinaigrette

SERVES 4

Prep time: 15 minutes

Cauliflower "rice" won't trick you into thinking that you're eating real rice, but it is delicious and satisfying in its own way. In this quick salad, it's studded with pomegranate seeds, hazelnuts, and grapes, and tossed with a bright dressing of fresh herbs and lemon.

SALAD

2 CUPS COARSELY CHOPPED CAULIFLOWER

½ CUP POMEGRANATE SEEDS

½ CUP RED GRAPES, CUT IN HALF

½ CUP HAZELNUTS, LIGHTLY TOASTED

2 CUPS GENTLY PACKED FRESH BABY SPINACH

FRESHLY GROUND PEPPER, FOR GARNISH

VINAIGRETTE

⅓ CUP FRESH BASIL

⅓ CUP FRESH CILANTRO

⅓ CUP FRESH PARSLEY

3 TABLESPOONS OLIVE OIL

JUICE OF 1 LEMON

½ TEASPOON SALT

1 GARLIC CLOVE, MINCED

1 TEASPOON HONEY

For the Salad:

1. Place the cauliflower in a food processor and pulse until chopped small (the size of grains of rice), but not pulverized or puréed. Transfer to a large salad bowl and set aside. Give the food processor a quick rinse and set aside.

2. To the cauliflower, add the pomegranate seeds, grapes, hazelnuts, and spinach and toss to combine.

For the Vinaigrette:

1. In the food processor combine the basil, cilantro, parsley, olive oil, lemon juice, salt, garlic, and honey, and process until well combined.

2. Drizzle the vinaigrette over the salad and toss to coat. Serve immediately, garnished with freshly ground pepper.

Roasted Butternut Squash Salad with Maple Vinaigrette

SERVES 4

Prep time: 10 minutes
Cook time: 20 minutes

Butternut squash is full of beta-carotene and other nutrients. Roasting it brings out an earthy natural sweetness that pairs beautifully with the maple vinaigrette. Serve this festive salad as part of a holiday meal or simply to celebrate a brisk fall day.

SALAD

3 CUPS BUTTERNUT SQUASH, CUT INTO 1-INCH DICE

1 TABLESPOON COCONUT OIL

½ TEASPOON SALT

10 CUPS GENTLY PACKED ARUGULA OR BABY SPINACH

½ RED ONION, THINLY SLICED

VINAIGRETTE

1 TABLESPOON MAPLE SYRUP

1 TABLESPOON RED WINE VINEGAR

1 TEASPOON DIJON MUSTARD

¼ TEASPOON SALT

⅛ TEASPOON PEPPER

2 TABLESPOONS OLIVE OIL

½ CUP CHOPPED PECANS, FOR GARNISH

FRESHLY GROUND PEPPER, FOR GARNISH

For the Salad:

1. Preheat the oven to 400°F.

2. On a large rimmed baking sheet, toss together the butternut squash and coconut oil until the squash is well coated. Sprinkle with the salt. Roast until tender and beginning to brown, about 20 minutes. Remove from the oven and let cool for about 5 minutes.

3. While the squash is roasting, place the arugula and red onion in a large salad bowl and toss to combine.

4. Add the squash to the arugula-onion mixture in the salad bowl and toss to combine.

For the Dressing:

1. In a small bowl, whisk together the maple syrup, vinegar, mustard, salt, and pepper. Whisking constantly, gradually add the olive oil in a thin stream. Whisk until well combined and emulsified.

2. Drizzle the vinaigrette over the salad and toss to coat well. Serve immediately, garnished with the pecans and freshly ground pepper.

Rainbow Root Veggie Slaw with Citrus-Cumin Vinaigrette

SERVES 4

Prep time: 10 minutes

This bright and crunchy slaw is a welcome change from the soggy, mayonnaise-heavy versions that are so common. Root veggies are shredded and tossed with a bright, mayo-less dressing of sherry vinegar, orange juice, and toasted cumin seeds. This salad is lovely eaten straightaway, but gets even better as it sits, so feel free to make it 30 minutes ahead of time, or more.

ZEST AND JUICE OF 1 ORANGE (ABOUT 1 TABLESPOON ZEST,
    ½ CUP JUICE)

1 TEASPOON TOASTED WHOLE CUMIN SEEDS

3 TABLESPOONS SHERRY VINEGAR

1 TABLESPOON OLIVE OIL

¾ TEASPOON SALT

½ TEASPOON PEPPER

½ TEASPOON HONEY

3 CARROTS, SHREDDED

2 BEETS, PEELED AND SHREDDED

1 CELERY ROOT, PEELED AND SHREDDED

1. Whisk together the orange zest, orange juice, cumin seeds, vinegar, oil, salt, pepper, and honey in a large salad bowl.

2. Add the carrots, beets, and celery root and toss to coat well.

3. Serve immediately or refrigerate, covered, for up to 3 days.

CHAPTER SIX

Entrées

Cauliflower Crust Pizza with Red Onions, Zucchini, and Cashew Cheese

SERVES 4

Prep time: 10 minutes
Cook time: 20 minutes

Thought you said farewell to pizza when you went Paleo? Think again. This grain-free pizza, on a crust made out of cauliflower, will rock your world. Here it gets a simple treatment with a quick tomato sauce, veggie toppings, and creamy cashew cheese, but you can top it with any of your favorite pizza toppings. This recipe has a fair number of ingredients, but this pizza is quick and easy to make.

CRUST

1 HEAD CAULIFLOWER, CORED AND CUT INTO SMALL FLORETS

2 TABLESPOONS ALMOND FLOUR

1 TABLESPOON COCONUT OIL

½ TEASPOON DRIED BASIL

½ TEASPOON DRIED OREGANO

¼ TEASPOON SALT

1 EGG, LIGHTLY BEATEN

COOKING SPRAY

SAUCE

2 TABLESPOONS COCONUT OIL

¼ ONION, DICED

3 GARLIC CLOVES, MINCED

ONE 28-OUNCE CAN DICED TOMATOES, WITH THEIR JUICE

1 TABLESPOON MINCED FRESH BASIL

1½ TEASPOONS SALT

½ TEASPOON PEPPER

½ RED ONION, SLICED VERY THIN

1 ZUCCHINI, SLICED VERY THIN

½ CUP CASHEW CHEESE (SEE PAGE 49)

For the Crust:

1. Place a pizza stone or baking sheet in the oven, and preheat the oven to 450°F.

2. Place the cauliflower in a food processor and pulse until it is in fine crumbs and looks a bit like snow. Transfer to a microwave-safe bowl, cover, and microwave on high for 4 minutes. Let cool, then transfer the cooked cauliflower to a clean dish towel and squeeze as much moisture out of it as you can.

3. In a medium bowl, combine the drained cauliflower with the almond flour, coconut oil, basil, oregano, and salt. Add the egg and mix well.

4. Place a piece of parchment paper on the counter and coat it with cooking spray. Turn the dough out onto the prepared parchment paper and, using your hands, pat it out into a 10-inch round pizza crust.

5. Using the parchment paper, transfer the crust onto the heated pizza stone or baking sheet. Bake until the crust begins to turn golden, about 6 minutes. Remove from the oven.

For the Sauce:

1. In a medium saucepan over medium-high heat, heat the oil. Add the diced onion and garlic and cook, stirring, until softened, about 5 minutes. Stir in the tomatoes and their juice, basil, salt, and pepper and bring to a boil. Reduce the heat to medium-low, cover, and simmer for 10 minutes.

2. Spoon the sauce onto the prebaked pizza crust and with the back of the spoon, spread it evenly out to the edges of the crust. Arrange the red onion and zucchini on top of the sauce.

3. Bake for about 15 minutes, until the sauce is bubbly and the vegetables are beginning to brown. Remove from the oven and drizzle with the cashew cheese. Cut into wedges and serve immediately.

Spaghetti (Squash) Carbonara

SERVES 4

Prep time: 5 minutes
Cook time: 20 minutes

Spaghetti squash is a delicious, nutritious, and fun substitute for pasta. Enjoy it here in a rich concoction of bacon and eggs.

1 SPAGHETTI SQUASH, HALVED AND SEEDED

6 EGGS

½ CUP COCONUT MILK

1 TABLESPOON ITALIAN SEASONING

1 TEASPOON DRIED PARSLEY

1 TEASPOON SALT

¼ TEASPOON GARLIC POWDER

¾ POUND BACON

1 TABLESPOON ARROWROOT POWDER

1 TABLESPOON GRASS-FED BUTTER OR LARD

1. Place the squash cut-side down on a plate and microwave for 10 minutes.

2. While the squash cooks, in a medium bowl, combine the eggs, coconut milk, Italian seasoning, parsley, salt, and garlic powder. Stir to mix well, and set aside.

3. In a large skillet over medium-high heat, cook the bacon until crisp, 6 to 8 minutes. Transfer the bacon to a paper towel–lined plate to drain. Cut the bacon into ¼-inch strips. Reserve the bacon grease in the skillet.

4. In the same skillet, whisk the arrowroot powder into the bacon grease and cook, stirring, for about 3 minutes.

5. Add the egg mixture to the skillet and cook, stirring frequently, for about 3 minutes until set but not dry. Transfer to a large serving bowl.

6. Scoop out the flesh of the squash and add it to the large serving bowl along with the bacon strips. Add the butter and stir to combine. Serve immediately.

Riceless Mushroom-Herb Risotto

Prep time: 10 minutes
Cook time: 15 minutes

Creamy risotto is a delicious treat, and this cauliflower version means that even devout Paleo dieters can once again indulge. Unlike the rice-based version, this one takes only 15 minutes to cook.

1 HEAD CAULIFLOWER, CUT INTO FLORETS

1 TABLESPOON COCONUT OIL

½ ONION, DICED

6 GARLIC CLOVES, MINCED

TWO 15-OUNCE CANS COCONUT MILK

1 TABLESPOON ARROWROOT POWDER DISSOLVED IN
    1 TABLESPOON WATER

1 TEASPOON SALT

½ TEASPOON PEPPER

¼ TEASPOON DRIED OREGANO

¼ TEASPOON DRIED BASIL

¼ TEASPOON DRIED MARJORAM

¼ TEASPOON DRIED THYME

1 POUND MUSHROOMS, SLICED THIN

2 TABLESPOONS CHOPPED FRESH CHIVES

1. Place the cauliflower in a food processor and pulse until minced into rice-size pieces. Set aside.

2. In a large stockpot over medium-high heat, heat the oil and add the onion and garlic. Cook, stirring frequently, until the onions are softened, about 5 minutes.

continued ▶

Riceless Mushroom-Herb Risotto *continued* ▶

3. Stir in the coconut milk, arrowroot mixture, salt, pepper, oregano, basil, marjoram, and thyme. Cook, whisking constantly, until the mixture begins to thicken, then add the mushrooms and chives. Cook, stirring, until the mushrooms begin to soften, about 2 minutes.

4. Stir in the minced cauliflower and cook, stirring constantly, until the cauliflower is soft but not mushy, about 5 minutes more. Serve hot.

Brazilian Garlic-Lime Shrimp

Prep time: 25 minutes (includes marinating time)
Cook time: 5 minutes

That nutritional powerhouse, garlic, makes a bold appearance in this quick, simple, but super flavorful shrimp dish. Serve it alongside cauliflower "rice" or sautéed chard.

2 POUNDS LARGE PEELED AND DEVEINED SHRIMP

2 TABLESPOONS FRESH LIME JUICE

½ CUP CHOPPED FRESH CILANTRO

8 GARLIC CLOVES, MINCED

½ TEASPOON SALT, DIVIDED

½ TEASPOON CRUSHED RED PEPPER FLAKES

2 TABLESPOONS COCONUT OIL

1. In a large nonreactive bowl, combine the shrimp with the lime juice, ¼ cup of the cilantro, half the minced garlic, ¼ teaspoon of the salt, and ¼ teaspoon of the red pepper flakes. Cover, refrigerate, and let marinate for about 20 minutes.

2. In a large, heavy skillet over medium-high heat, heat the oil. When the oil is very hot, add the shrimp, along with the marinade and the remaining garlic. Cook, stirring frequently, until the shrimp are pink and cooked through, about 5 minutes.

3. Remove from the heat and stir in the remaining ¼ cup of cilantro, ¼ teaspoon of salt, and ¼ teaspoon of crushed red pepper flakes. Serve immediately.

Thai Shrimp Curry

SERVES 4

Prep time: 10 minutes
Cook time: 15 minutes

This is a super easy recipe and all of the ingredients can be substituted. Don't want to splurge on prawns? Use chicken instead. Don't have broccoli? Substitute cauliflower or zucchini. Don't like cilantro? It's just as good with fresh basil. You can even replace the spices with a tablespoon or two of Thai curry paste.

1 SHALLOT

3 GARLIC CLOVES

1-INCH PIECE OF PEELED FRESH GINGER, HALVED

1 TEASPOON GROUND CORIANDER

1½ TEASPOONS GROUND CUMIN

⅛ TEASPOON GROUND NUTMEG

¾ TEASPOON GROUND TURMERIC

¼ TEASPOON FENNEL SEED

⅛ TEASPOON CAYENNE PEPPER

3 TABLESPOONS FISH SAUCE

2 KAFFIR LIME LEAVES OR 1 TEASPOON LIME ZEST

1 TABLESPOON PALM SUGAR

ONE 16-OUNCE CAN COCONUT MILK

1 TABLESPOON TOMATO PASTE

1 TABLESPOON COCONUT BUTTER

2 CARROTS, DICED

1 HEAD BROCCOLI, CUT INTO SMALL FLORETS

1 RED BELL PEPPER, DICED

1 POUND PEELED AND DEVEINED PRAWNS

½ CUP CHOPPED FRESH CILANTRO

JUICE OF ½ LIME

1. In a food processor, combine the shallot, garlic, ginger, coriander, cumin, nutmeg, turmeric, fennel seed, cayenne, and fish sauce, and pulse until finely chopped and paste-like.

2. Transfer the mixture to a large stockpot and add the kaffir lime leaves, palm sugar, coconut milk, tomato paste, and coconut butter. Bring to a boil, stirring frequently, over medium-high heat.

3. Reduce the heat to medium-low and add the carrots, broccoli, and bell pepper. Cook for 6 to 8 minutes, until the vegetables are tender. Add the prawns and cook until they are pink and cooked through, about 3 minutes.

4. Just before serving, stir in the cilantro and lime juice. Serve hot.

Pan-Seared Salmon with Tropical Salsa

SERVES 4

Prep time: 10 minutes
Cook time: 8 minutes

This salmon dish gives you the health benefits of salmon with its high dose of omega-3 fatty acids, plus the deliciousness and nutrition of both mango and avocado. The best thing is that it takes barely 10 minutes to prep and even less than that to cook.

SALSA

2 RIPE MANGOS, DICED

½ CUP FINELY DICED RED ONION

1 AVOCADO, DICED

1 JALAPEÑO PEPPER, SEEDED AND FINELY DICED

¼ CUP MINCED FRESH CILANTRO

2 TABLESPOONS COCONUT OIL

¾ TEASPOON SALT

½ TEASPOON PEPPER

JUICE FROM 1 LIME

SALMON

2 TABLESPOONS COCONUT OIL

4 FRESH WILD SALMON FILLETS (ABOUT 6 OUNCES EACH)

½ TEASPOON SALT

¼ TEASPOON PEPPER

For the Salsa:

In a medium bowl, combine the mangos, onion, avocado, jalapeño, cilantro, coconut oil, salt, pepper and lime juice, and stir to mix well. Set aside.

For the Salmon:

1. In a large skillet over high heat, heat the coconut oil. Add the salmon, skin-side down, and immediately reduce the heat to medium-low. Season the salmon with the salt and pepper. Gently press each piece of salmon down with a spatula to ensure that the skin crisps evenly. Cook until the crispy skin releases from the surface of the skillet, about 5 to 6 minutes. Turn the salmon fillets over and sear the other side for about 30 seconds.

2. Transfer the salmon fillets to serving plates and top each with a generous spoonful of salsa. Serve immediately.

Pan-Seared Trout with Cherry Tomatoes and Bacon

SERVES 4

Prep time: 5 minutes
Cook time: 10 minutes

In this dish, you get lots of protein and the heart-healthy benefits of fish, plus the mouthwatering flavor of smoky bacon. Serve this with oven-roasted Brussels sprouts for a satisfying meal.

4 SLICES BACON

1 PINT CHERRY TOMATOES, HALVED

1 GARLIC CLOVE, MINCED

1 TEASPOON SALT

1 TEASPOON PEPPER

1 TABLESPOON MINCED FRESH THYME

4 TROUT FILLETS (ABOUT 6 OUNCES EACH)

2 TEASPOONS COCONUT OIL

4 LEMON WEDGES

1. In a medium skillet over medium-high heat, cook the bacon, turning once, until crisp, 5 to 7 minutes.

2. Transfer the bacon strips to a paper towel–lined plate to drain and cool, then crumble the bacon. Drain off all but about 1 tablespoon of the bacon fat from the pan.

3. Add the cherry tomatoes, garlic, ½ teaspoon of the salt, and ½ teaspoon of the pepper to the bacon fat in the pan and cook, stirring, until the tomatoes just begin to break down, about 3 minutes. Remove from the heat, and stir in the crumbled bacon and the thyme. Set aside.

4. In a large nonstick skillet over medium-high heat, heat the coconut oil. Sprinkle the fish fillets with the remaining $\frac{1}{2}$ teaspoon of salt and $\frac{1}{2}$ teaspoon of pepper. Add the trout fillets to the pan (you may need to cook the fish in two batches to avoid overcrowding). Cook the fish, turning once, until it is cooked through and flakes easily with a fork, 2 to 3 minutes per side.

5. Transfer the fish fillets to serving plates. Serve topped with the cherry tomato mixture, with lemon wedges on the side.

Baked Cod with Lemon and Herbs

SERVES 4

Prep time: 5 minutes
Cook time: 20 minutes

This straightforward recipe allows a good piece of delicious cod to really shine. You could also substitute other white fish, such as sole or snapper. Serve it alongside roasted or pan-seared broccoli or Brussels sprouts.

4 COD FILLETS (ABOUT 6 OUNCES EACH)
1½ TABLESPOONS LEMON JUICE
1 TABLESPOON COCONUT OIL
2 CLOVES GARLIC, CRUSHED AND MINCED
1 TEASPOON MINCED FRESH THYME
1 TEASPOON SALT
½ TEASPOON PEPPER
½ TEASPOON SWEET PAPRIKA

1. Preheat the oven to 400°F.

2. Arrange the fish fillets in a 9-by-13-inch shallow baking dish. Over the top, sprinkle the lemon juice, coconut oil, garlic, thyme, salt, pepper, and paprika.

3. Bake for 15 to 20 minutes, until the fish is opaque and flakes easily with a fork. Serve hot.

Tangy Chicken Piccata

Prep time: 10 minutes
Cook time: 15 minutes

This classic Italian dish is usually made with cheese and flour. This recipe uses almond flour and skips the cheese, but still delivers all the tangy, delicious flavor you want in a chicken piccata.

2 BONELESS, SKINLESS CHICKEN BREASTS

1 EGG

2 TABLESPOONS WATER

½ CUP ALMOND FLOUR

1 TEASPOON SALT

½ TEASPOON BLACK PEPPER

¼ TEASPOON CAYENNE PEPPER

1 TABLESPOON CHICKEN BROTH

JUICE OF 1 LEMON

½ CUP WHITE WINE

1 TABLESPOON CAPERS, DRAINED

1 TABLESPOON MINCED FRESH PARSLEY

1. Preheat the oven to 400°F.

2. Halve the 2 chicken breasts horizontally so that you have 4 thin fillets. If desired, pound the chicken fillets between two pieces of plastic wrap to ¼-inch thickness.

3. In a shallow bowl, whisk together the egg and water. In another shallow bowl, combine the almond flour, salt, black pepper, and cayenne. Dredge the chicken fillets first in the egg and then in the flour mixture.

continued ▶

4. In a large, oven-safe skillet over high heat, heat the oil. Add the chicken to the hot pan and cook for about 3 minutes, until one side is nicely browned. Turn the chicken over and cook on the second side until golden brown, about 3 minutes.

5. Transfer the skillet to the oven and bake until cooked through, about 5 minutes.

6. Transfer the chicken to serving plates. To the skillet, add the chicken broth, lemon juice, and wine and cook over medium heat, stirring up the flavorful brown bits on the bottom of the pan. Simmer the sauce until it is reduced by about half, about 2 minutes. Stir in the capers and spoon the sauce over the chicken breasts. Serve immediately, garnished with parsley.

Tortilla-less Chicken Enchiladas

SERVES 4

Prep time: 5 minutes
Cook time: 25 minutes

A great enchilada is determined by its sauce, and this one easily measures up. You won't even miss the tortillas. Use leftover roasted or rotisserie chicken for a quick and satisfying meal.

2 TABLESPOONS COCONUT OIL

1 ONION, FINELY DICED

ONE 16-OUNCE CAN TOMATO PURÉE

4 GARLIC CLOVES, MINCED

2 TABLESPOONS CHILI POWDER

½ TEASPOON GROUND CUMIN

½ TEASPOON DRIED OREGANO

½ TEASPOON SALT

1 POUND COOKED, SHREDDED CHICKEN

1 AVOCADO, SLICED, FOR GARNISH

¼ CUP CHOPPED FRESH CILANTRO, FOR GARNISH

1 LIME, CUT INTO WEDGES, FOR GARNISH

½ CUP CASHEW CHEESE (PAGE 49), FOR GARNISH (OPTIONAL)

1. Preheat the oven to 375°F.

2. In a large skillet over medium-high heat, heat the coconut oil. Add the onion and cook, stirring frequently, until softened, about 5 minutes. Stir in the tomato purée, garlic, chili powder, cumin, oregano, and salt and bring to a boil. Reduce the heat to medium-low and simmer for 15 minutes, stirring occasionally.

continued ▶

3. Purée the sauce until smooth using an immersion blender, or purée in batches using a food processor or countertop blender.

4. Place the chicken in a 9-by-13-inch shallow baking dish and pour the sauce over the top. Cover tightly with foil and bake for 10 minutes, until hot and bubbling.

5. Serve immediately, garnished with avocado, cilantro, lime wedges, and cashew cheese, if using.

Baked Ginger Chicken Thighs

Prep time: 5 minutes
Cook time: 25 minutes

This easy dish is tangy, sweet, and all-around delicious. Best of all, it's the kind of dish that's loved equally by kids and adults.

1 BUNCH SCALLIONS, TRIMMED AND CUT INTO THIRDS

2 GARLIC CLOVES, MINCED

8 QUARTER-SIZE SLICES OF FRESH PEELED GINGER

3 TABLESPOONS RICE VINEGAR

3 TABLESPOONS COCONUT OIL

2 TABLESPOONS FISH SAUCE

2 TABLESPOONS HONEY

½ TEASPOON TOASTED SESAME OIL

1½ TEASPOONS SALT

½ TEASPOON PEPPER

1 POUND BONELESS CHICKEN THIGHS

1. Preheat the oven to 400°F.

2. Combine the scallions, garlic, ginger, vinegar, coconut oil, fish sauce, honey, sesame oil, salt, and pepper in a food processor and process until smooth.

3. Arrange the chicken, skin-side up, in a single layer in a shallow 9-by-13-inch baking dish. Pour the sauce over the chicken, turning to coat.

4. Bake until cooked through, about 25 minutes. Serve hot.

Creamy Green Chile Chicken

SERVES 4

Prep time: 5 minutes
Cook time: 25 minutes

Almonds and almond milk give this simple chicken dish a rich, creamy mouth-feel and a flavor that is out of this world. Using chicken breast tenders cuts down on the prep time, but you could use whole boneless chicken breasts and cut them into fillets yourself.

2 CUPS UNSWEETENED ALMOND MILK

½ CUP CHICKEN BROTH

¾ CUP CHOPPED, SEEDED FRESH NEW MEXICAN GREEN CHILES

3 GREEN ONIONS, SLICED, WHITE AND GREEN PARTS SEPARATED

3 TABLESPOONS SLIVERED ALMONDS, TOASTED

1 GARLIC CLOVE, THINLY SLICED

¾ TEASPOON SALT, DIVIDED

1½ POUNDS CHICKEN BREAST TENDERS

1 TABLESPOON COCONUT OIL

1 TABLESPOON SESAME SEEDS, TOASTED

1. In a medium saucepan over medium-high heat, add the almond milk, broth, green chiles, the white parts of the green onions, almonds, garlic, and ¼ teaspoon of the salt, and stir to combine. Bring to a boil. Lower the heat to low and simmer until reduced to half, about 20 minutes.

2. Meanwhile, in a large nonstick skillet over medium-high heat, heat the coconut oil. Sprinkle the remaining ½ teaspoon of salt on the chicken and add the chicken to the pan. Cook until browned on one side, about 2 minutes, then turn over and cook until browned on the second side, about 2 minutes more.

3. Using an immersion blender or a countertop blender, purée the green chile sauce until smooth.

4. Transfer the sauce to the skillet with the chicken and bring to a simmer. Cook for 5 minutes, until the chicken is thoroughly cooked. Serve the chicken hot, garnished with the reserved green parts of the green onions and the sesame seeds.

Quick and Easy Pork Chops with Sautéed Mushrooms

Prep time: 5 minutes
Cook time: 25 minutes

An easy-to-make mushroom sauce dresses up pork chops for a satisfying meal that can be on your table in no time. Serve this dish alongside mashed cauliflower for a real meat-and-potatoes-style meal.

4 BONE-IN, CENTER-CUT PORK CHOPS

1 TEASPOON SALT

½ TEASPOON PEPPER

1 TABLESPOON COCONUT OIL

1 ONION, SLICED

3 GARLIC CLOVES, MINCED

1 POUND MUSHROOMS (BUTTON OR CREMINI, OR A MIXTURE), SLICED

2 TEASPOONS MINCED FRESH ROSEMARY OR ½ TEASPOON DRIED ROSEMARY

½ CUP CHICKEN BROTH

1. Season the pork chops with the salt and pepper.

2. In a large skillet over medium-high heat, heat the oil. Add pork chops and cook until nicely browned on one side, about 3 minutes. Turn over the pork chops and cook until the second side is nicely browned, about 3 minutes more. Remove the chops from the pan.

3. Add the onion and garlic to the skillet, reduce the heat to medium, and cook, stirring frequently, until softened, about 5 minutes. Add the mushrooms and rosemary, cooking until the mushrooms are tender, 5 to 7 minutes.

continued ▶

Quick and Easy Pork Chops with Sautéed Mushrooms *continued* ▶

4. Add the broth and bring to a simmer. Return the pork chops to the pan, cover, reduce the heat to medium-low, and simmer until the pork is cooked through, about 8 minutes.

5. Serve the pork chops immediately with the mushrooms spooned over the top.

Spicy Chinese Beef in Lettuce Cups

SERVES 4

Prep time: 10 minutes
Cook time: 15 minutes

This spicy meat mixture makes a tasty filling for crisp lettuce leaves. Coconut aminos is a soy-free substitute for soy sauce. Made by aging raw coconut tree sap, it is, like soy sauce, dark, rich, salty, and full of umami, or savory goodness. You can find it at health food stores, or a natural foods store like Whole Foods.

2 TABLESPOONS COCONUT OIL

1 ONION, FINELY DICED

1 POUND GROUND BEEF

1 TEASPOON SALT

2 GARLIC CLOVES, MINCED

2 TABLESPOONS MINCED, PEELED FRESH GINGER

2 TABLESPOONS COCONUT AMINOS

1 TABLESPOON RICE VINEGAR

1 TABLESPOON SESAME OIL

1 TABLESPOON ALMOND BUTTER

2 TEASPOONS WATER

2 TEASPOONS HONEY

2 TEASPOONS ASIAN CHILI PASTE

½ CUP SLICED GREEN ONIONS

½ CUP DICED WATER CHESTNUTS

12 LETTUCE LEAVES

¼ CUP CASHEWS, FOR GARNISH

continued ▶

1. In a large skillet over medium-high heat, heat the oil. Add the onion and cook, stirring frequently, until softened, about 5 minutes. Add the beef and salt and cook, stirring and breaking up the meat with a spatula, until browned, about 5 minutes. Spoon off any excess fat.

2. In a small bowl, whisk together the garlic, ginger, coconut aminos, rice vinegar, sesame oil, almond butter, water, honey, and chili paste until smooth. Add this mixture to the beef and cook, stirring, until heated through, 3 or 4 minutes.

3. Stir in the green onions and water chestnuts and cook until heated through, about 2 minutes more.

4. Serve scooped into lettuce leaves and garnished with cashews.

Lemon-Rosemary Seared Steak with Asparagus and Mushrooms

Prep time: 5 minutes
Cook time: 20 minutes

Seared steak with tender sautéed asparagus and mushrooms is a quick, delicious, and elegant meal. In this dish, the flavors of lemon zest, rosemary, and garlic shine.

1½ POUNDS FLANK STEAK, 1-INCH THICK

4 GARLIC CLOVES, MINCED

1 TABLESPOON FRESH ROSEMARY LEAVES, MINCED

1 TEASPOON SALT

½ TEASPOON PEPPER

2 TABLESPOONS COCONUT OIL

1 ONION, THINLY SLICED LENGTHWISE

1 POUND ASPARAGUS, TRIMMED AND CUT INTO 2-INCH PIECES

1 POUND BUTTON OR CREMINI MUSHROOMS, SLICED

1 TEASPOON GRATED LEMON ZEST

1. Using a sharp knife, make ⅛-inch-deep cuts in the steak in a diamond pattern on both sides. Spread half of the garlic and half of the rosemary onto the steak on both sides, and then sprinkle with ½ teaspoon of the salt and ¼ teaspoon of the pepper.

continued ▶

2. In a large skillet over medium-high heat, heat 1 tablespoon of the coconut oil. When the pan is very hot, add the steak and cook about 4 minutes per side (longer if you prefer it more done than medium-rare). Transfer the steak to a cutting board, cover with foil, and let rest for at least 5 minutes.

3. Heat the remaining tablespoon of oil in the skillet and add the onion. Cook, stirring frequently, until the onion begins to soften, about 3 minutes. Add the remaining garlic and cook another 2 minutes.

4. Stir in the asparagus, mushrooms, and the remaining ½ teaspoon of salt, and the remaining ¼ teaspoon of pepper and cook, stirring frequently, until the mushrooms are soft and the asparagus is crisp-tender, about 5 minutes. Add the lemon zest and the remaining rosemary.

5. To serve, slice the steak across the grain into ⅛-inch-thick slices and serve with the vegetables.

Thai Beef Meatballs

SERVES 4

Prep time: 10 minutes
Cook time: 20 minutes

These simple meatballs are flavored with classic Thai ingredients like chiles, garlic, basil, and fish sauce. Serve them with roasted, grilled, or steamed vegetables, or on top of spaghetti squash or other vegetable "noodles."

1 TABLESPOON COCONUT OIL, MELTED

2 EGGS, LIGHTLY BEATEN

½ CUP ALMOND FLOUR

1 ROASTED RED THAI CHILE PEPPER, SEEDED AND CHOPPED
   (ABOUT ⅓ CUP)

¼ CUP FISH SAUCE

3 GARLIC CLOVES, MINCED

2 TEASPOONS ASIAN CHILI PASTE

½ CUP CHOPPED FRESH BASIL

ZEST OF 1 LIME

1½ POUNDS GROUND BEEF

1. Preheat the oven 400°F. Brush a large baking sheet with a bit of the coconut oil.

2. In a large bowl, combine the eggs, almond flour, red pepper, fish sauce, garlic, chili paste, basil, and lime zest and whisk to combine. Add the beef and mix well, using your hands if necessary.

3. Form the meat mixture into 1-inch balls and place them on the prepared baking sheet. Brush the tops of the meatballs with the remaining coconut oil.

4. Bake until browned on top and cooked through, about 20 minutes.
Serve hot.

Spiced Lamb Kebabs

Prep time: 15 minutes
Cook time: 10 minutes

Loaded with herbs and spices, these kebabs are very satisfying. If you prefer, substitute grass-fed ground beef for the lamb. If using wooden skewers, soak them in water for 30 minutes first. Serve with a refreshing cucumber and tomato salad for a quick and delicious meal.

2 SHALLOTS

2 CLOVES GARLIC

3 QUARTER-SIZE SLICES OF FRESH PEELED GINGER

ZEST AND JUICE OF 1 LEMON

½ CUP FRESH CILANTRO LEAVES

4 SPRIGS FRESH MINT

1 TEASPOON GARAM MASALA

¾ TEASPOON KOSHER SALT

½ TEASPOON PEPPER

1 POUND GROUND LAMB

1 TABLESPOON HONEY

½ TEASPOON BAKING SODA

1. In a food processor, process the shallots, garlic, ginger, lemon zest, cilantro, mint, garam masala, salt, and pepper until minced.

2. Transfer the shallot mixture to a large bowl and add the lamb, honey, and baking soda. Mix with your hands until well combined, 2 or 3 minutes.

3. Divide the meat mixture into 8 equal portions and roll each into a cylinder. Press each portion onto a skewer, flattening it to about ¼-inch thick, and squeeze to seal it onto the stick. Repeat to form all of the kebabs.

4. Oil a grill or grill pan and heat to medium. Grill the skewers for about 2 minutes; then rotate them 45 degrees and cook for another 2 minutes. Turn the skewers 45 degrees more and cook 2 additional minutes, then rotate another 45 degrees and cook until the meat is thoroughly cooked, 2 to 3 minutes. Serve hot.

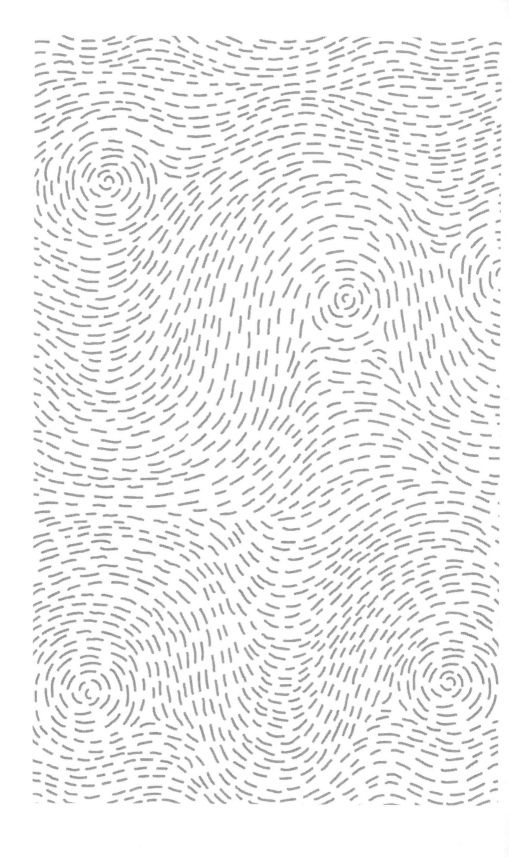

CHAPTER SEVEN

Desserts

Tropical Sweet Bites

MAKES 16 BARS

Prep time: 25 minutes

Dried pineapple is naturally extremely sweet, so there's no need for any additional sweetener in this recipe. Keep these energy-packed goodies in the fridge for any time you need a quick pick-me-up or a sweet taste of the tropics.

2 CUPS UNSWEETENED DRIED PINEAPPLE

⅔ CUP HOT WATER

2 CUPS RAW CASHEWS

½ CUP UNSWEETENED COCONUT FLAKES

1 TEASPOON LEMON ZEST

¼ TEASPOON SALT

1. Line an 8-by-8-inch baking pan with parchment paper.

2. In a medium bowl, cover the pineapple with the hot water. Let soak for about 5 minutes and drain, discarding the liquid.

3. In a food processor, combine the pineapple, cashews, coconut flakes, lemon zest, and salt, and process until the mixture is finely ground and forms a sticky batter.

4. Transfer the mixture to the prepared baking pan and smooth it out until even. Freeze until firm, 10 to 15 minutes. Cut into 16 bars and serve immediately, or store, covered, in the refrigerator for up to 1 week.

Spiced Apple Pie Bites

MAKES ABOUT 24 BALLS

Prep time: 10 minutes

These healthy little bites taste just like apple pie, but they are 100 percent grain-free, nut-free, and dairy-free.

1 CUP DRIED FIGS

1 CUP UNSWEETENED APPLESAUCE

½ TABLESPOON GROUND CINNAMON

¼ CUP ALMOND FLOUR

¼ CUP COCONUT FLOUR

1 CUP WALNUTS

½ CUP ALMONDS

CINNAMON COATING

½ CUP ALMONDS

½ TABLESPOON GROUND CINNAMON

1. Place the figs, applesauce, and cinnamon in a food processor and process until smooth. Transfer the mixture to a large bowl and stir in the almond flour and coconut flour.

2. Place the walnuts and almonds in the food processor and pulse until coarsely ground. Stir them into the fig mixture in the bowl. Set in the refrigerator to chill while you make the cinnamon coating.

For the Cinnamon Coating:

1. Place the almonds and cinnamon in the food processor and pulse until finely ground. Transfer the mixture to a small bowl.

2. Form the fig mixture into 1-inch balls and roll them in the cinnamon coating. Serve immediately or chill in the refrigerator until ready to serve.

Broiled Figs with Caramel

SERVES 4 TO 6

Prep time: 5 minutes
Cook time: 15 minutes

This simple dessert has just a few ingredients, but tastes sinfully decadent. Try it with apples or peaches, depending on what's in season.

CARAMEL

1 CUP COCONUT MILK

½ CUP HONEY

2 TABLESPOONS COCONUT PALM SUGAR

FIGS

12 FRESH, RIPE FIGS, TRIMMED AND HALVED

1 TABLESPOON COCONUT OIL

¼ TEASPOON GROUND CINNAMON

Preheat the broiler to high.

For the Caramel:

In a medium saucepan over medium-high heat, combine the coconut milk, honey, and coconut palm sugar. Bring almost to a boil, stirring frequently. Cook, stirring, until the sauce becomes very thick and dark, about 10 minutes.

For the Figs:

1. Place the figs, cut-side up, on a baking sheet and brush with the coconut oil. Place under the broiler and cook until they begin to caramelize, 3 to 4 minutes.

2. Remove from the broiler and place on serving plates. Drizzle with the caramel and sprinkle with the cinnamon.

Vanilla-Coconut Macaroons

Prep time: 5 minutes
Cook time: 15 minutes

These simple cookies deliver big, bold coconut flavor. They are just the thing when you need a little snack to accompany a cup of tea in the afternoon, but are sweet enough to act as a satisfying dessert after a festive dinner, as well.

2 EGG WHITES
¼ CUP MAPLE SYRUP
½ TEASPOON VANILLA EXTRACT
¼ TEASPOON SEA SALT
2 CUPS UNSWEETENED, SHREDDED COCONUT

1. Preheat the oven to 350°F. Line a baking sheet with parchment paper.

2. Whisk together the egg whites, maple syrup, vanilla, and salt until frothy. Stir in the coconut.

3. Scoop the dough onto the prepared baking sheet using a small cookie scoop or melon baller.

4. Bake until the bottoms and edges turn golden brown, about 12 to 15 minutes. Remove from the oven and let cool in the pan. Serve warm or at room temperature.

Sunflower Seed–Butter Cookies

MAKES ABOUT 12 COOKIES

Prep time: 10 minutes
Cook time: 12 minutes

These simple cookies have only five ingredients, but they are full of flavor. Hemp seeds are a great source of easily digestible protein, and they may also be the only edible source of gamma linoleic acid, a healthy omega-6 fat that supports anti-inflammatory hormone function. You can buy hemp seeds at health food stores or a natural foods store like Whole Foods.

⅔ CUP SUNFLOWER SEED BUTTER
⅔ CUP HEMP SEEDS
¼ CUP HONEY
1 TEASPOON VANILLA EXTRACT
1 EGG WHITE, AT ROOM TEMPERATURE

1. Preheat the oven to 350°F. Line a rimmed baking sheet with parchment paper.

2. In a medium bowl, stir together the sunflower seed butter, hemp seeds, honey, and vanilla.

3. In a separate medium bowl, with an electric mixer set on high speed, beat the egg white until very fluffy. Add the sunflower seed butter mixture and stir with the mixer until smooth and well combined.

4. Drop the mixture by tablespoonfuls onto the prepared baking sheet. Bake the cookies until they begin to turn golden and crack a bit, about 10 to 12 minutes. Let them cool on the pan. Serve warm or at room temperature.

Cinnamon-Glazed Almond Cookies

MAKES ABOUT 24 COOKIES

Prep time: 10 minutes
Cook time: 20 minutes

The combination of almond flour and coconut flour helps hold these cookies together. The cinnamon glaze makes them completely addictive.

COOKIES

2½ CUPS ALMOND FLOUR, PLUS MORE FOR DUSTING

¼ CUP COCONUT FLOUR

2 TEASPOONS BAKING POWDER

½ TEASPOON GROUND CINNAMON

¼ CUP COCONUT OIL

1 TABLESPOON HONEY

1 TEASPOON VANILLA EXTRACT

2 EGGS, LIGHTLY BEATEN

GLAZE

2 TABLESPOONS HONEY

1 TABLESPOON COCONUT BUTTER, MELTED

1 TABLESPOON GROUND CINNAMON

For the Cookies:

1. Preheat the oven to 350°F. Line a large rimmed baking sheet with parchment paper.

2. In a large bowl, combine the almond flour, coconut flour, baking powder, and cinnamon. Add the coconut oil, honey, vanilla, and eggs, and stir until it forms a soft dough.

continued ▶

3. Dust the work surface with a bit of almond flour and press the dough out to about ½-inch thickness. Using a 2½-inch round cutter, cut the dough into circles and arrange them on the prepared baking sheet. Bake for about 10 minutes.

For the Glaze:

1. In a small bowl, stir together the honey, coconut butter, and cinnamon.

2. Take the cookies out of the oven (leave the oven on) and brush them all over with the glaze. Return to the oven and bake for another 10 minutes.

3. Remove from the oven and drizzle with more glaze, if desired. Cool on a wire rack and serve warm or at room temperature.

Nutty Pecan Shortbread

Prep time: 10 minutes
Cook time: 20 minutes

These rich, crumbly cookies are bursting with pecan flavor. Serve them with hot tea for a relaxing treat.

6 TABLESPOONS ALMOND FLOUR
6 TABLESPOONS COCONUT PALM SUGAR
½ CUP ARROWROOT POWDER
¼ TEASPOON SALT
1 TEASPOON BAKING SODA
1 EGG
⅓ CUP COCONUT BUTTER
1 TEASPOON VANILLA EXTRACT
ZEST OF ½ LEMON
½ CUP TOASTED PECANS, CHOPPED

1. Preheat the oven to 350°F. Line a large baking sheet with parchment paper.

2. In a food processor, combine the almond flour, coconut sugar, arrowroot powder, salt, and baking soda and process to a fine powder.

3. Add the egg, coconut butter, vanilla, and lemon zest, and process until the mixture becomes a thick dough. Add the pecans and pulse a few times.

4. Place the dough on a piece of plastic wrap and form it into a ball, then flatten the ball into a 1-inch-thick disk. Wrap the plastic wrap around the dough and put in the freezer for about 10 minutes.

5. Place the dough between two pieces of parchment paper, and with a rolling pin, roll it to about a ¼-inch thickness.

continued ▶

Nutty Pecan Shortbread *continued* ▶

6. Cut the dough into whatever shapes you like (circles or squares) and arrange them on the prepared baking sheet with ⅛ inch between.

7. Bake until the shortbread cookies just begin to turn golden brown, about 17 minutes. Transfer to a wire rack to cool. Serve at room temperature.

Chocolate Chip Cookies Paleofied

Prep time: 10 minutes
Cook time: 10 minutes

Certain things simply defy being given up, no matter what the promised health benefits. Chocolate chip cookies certainly fall into that category. These are every bit as delicious as the classic cookies your mom used to make, but they are grain-free and sweetened with maple syrup.

1 TABLESPOON COCONUT OIL, MELTED, PLUS MORE FOR THE
     BAKING SHEET
1½ CUPS ALMOND FLOUR
¼ TEASPOON BAKING SODA
¼ TEASPOON SALT
½ TEASPOON VANILLA EXTRACT
½ CUP MAPLE SYRUP
1 EGG
½ CUP DARK CHOCOLATE CHIPS

1. Preheat the oven to 350°F. Coat a large baking sheet with a bit of coconut oil.

2. In a medium bowl, combine the almond flour, baking soda, and salt. Set aside.

3. In a large bowl, combine the 1 tablespoon of coconut oil, vanilla, maple syrup, and egg, and stir to combine. Add the almond flour mixture and mix well. Stir in the chocolate chips.

4. Drop the cookies by spoonfuls onto the prepared baking sheet. Bake until the edges begin to turn golden brown, about 10 minutes. Transfer to a wire rack to cool. Serve warm or at room temperature.

Strawberry Shortcakes with Whipped Coconut Cream

SERVES 8

Prep time: 10 minutes
Cook time: 20 minutes

If you can't find coconut cream, you can make your own. Chill a 15-ounce can of full-fat coconut milk in the refrigerator overnight. Without shaking the can or turning it over, remove the lid of the can. The cream will have risen to the top. Scoop off this thick layer, discarding the watery liquid below or reserving it for another use.

SHORTCAKES

2 CUPS ALMOND FLOUR

½ TEASPOON BAKING SODA

1 TEASPOON GROUND CINNAMON

3 TABLESPOONS COCONUT OIL, CHILLED

2 EGGS

2 TABLESPOONS HONEY

1 TEASPOON VANILLA EXTRACT

1 POUND FRESH STRAWBERRIES, SLICED

WHIPPED COCONUT CREAM

1 CUP COCONUT CREAM

2 TABLESPOONS HONEY OR MAPLE SYRUP

½ TEASPOON VANILLA EXTRACT

For the Shortcakes:

1. Preheat the oven to 350°F. Line a baking sheet with parchment paper.

2. In a food processor, combine the almond flour, baking soda, and cinnamon. Add the coconut oil and pulse until the mixture resembles coarse meal.

3. In a small bowl, whisk together the eggs, honey, and vanilla. Add the egg mixture to the flour mixture in the food processor and process just until the dough comes together in a ball.

4. Drop the dough onto the prepared baking sheet in 8 equal portions, leaving 2 inches of space between them. Bake until golden brown, 15 to 20 minutes.

For the Whipped Coconut Cream:

1. In a large bowl, using an electric mixer on high speed, whip the coconut cream until it becomes very fluffy and forms soft peaks. Add the honey and vanilla and beat just to incorporate.

2. Remove the cakes from the oven and let them cool for a few minutes on a wire rack. Split each horizontally.

3. To serve, top the lower half of a shortcake with sliced strawberries and a large dollop of coconut cream, then place the other half on top. Repeat with the remaining shortcakes, strawberries, and coconut cream. Serve immediately.

Berry Cobbler

Prep time: 5 minutes
Cook time: 25 minutes

This quick cobbler is a delicious dessert in the summer when berries are at their peak, but you can substitute thawed frozen berries anytime of year if you like.

3 CUPS FRESH BERRIES (STRAWBERRIES, BLACKBERRIES, RASPBERRIES, BLUEBERRIES, OR A COMBINATION)
1 TABLESPOON HONEY
1 EGG, LIGHTLY BEATEN
1½ CUPS ALMOND FLOUR
2 TABLESPOONS COCONUT OIL
½ TEASPOON GROUND CINNAMON

1. Preheat the oven to 375°F.

2. Place the berries in a 9-inch pie dish and drizzle the honey over the top.

3. In a small bowl, combine the egg, almond flour, coconut oil, and cinnamon, and stir to mix into a crumbly topping. Using your hands, crumble the topping mixture over the berries in an even layer.

4. Bake until lightly browned and crisp on top, about 25 minutes. Serve hot.

Maple-Tapioca Pudding

Prep time: 20 minutes
Cook time: 5 minutes

This simple pudding, sweetened with a touch of maple syrup, is humble comfort food at its best. Easy and quick to make, it will warm the belly and the heart.

3 TABLESPOONS DRY TAPIOCA PEARLS
¾ CUP WATER
1 EGG, SEPARATED
2 TABLESPOONS MAPLE SYRUP
¾ CUP COCONUT MILK
½ TEASPOON VANILLA EXTRACT

1. In a small saucepan, stir together the tapioca pearls and water. Let sit to allow the tapioca to soften, about 15 minutes.

2. Meanwhile, in a medium bowl, whisk the egg white until soft peaks form. Mix in the maple syrup. Set aside.

3. Set the tapioca and water mixture over medium heat and whisk in the coconut milk and egg yolk. Cook, whisking constantly, until the mixture thickens, 3 or 4 minutes.

4. Remove from the heat and stir in the vanilla. Fold the warm tapioca mixture into the egg white mixture. Serve warm, or let cool to room temperature, then refrigerate and serve chilled.

Dark Chocolate Coconut Bark

MAKES 16 PIECES

Prep time: 20 minutes
Cook time: 5 minutes

This recipe is ridiculously easy and so delicious. Be sure to use unrefined coconut oil for the right texture.

2 OUNCES DARK CHOCOLATE, CHOPPED
1 CUP UNREFINED COCONUT OIL
¼ CUP FLAKED COCONUT
¼ CUP SLIVERED ALMONDS

1. Line an 8-by-8-inch baking pan with parchment paper.

2. Place the chocolate in the top of a double boiler set over simmering water. Cook until the chocolate begins to melt, 3 or 4 minutes. Remove the pot from the heat and stir in the coconut oil. Continue to stir until the chocolate is completely melted and the mixture is well combined. Stir in the coconut and almonds.

3. Pour the mixture into the prepared baking pan and chill in the freezer until the chocolate is solid, about 15 minutes.

4. Cut into 2-inch squares, wrap in plastic wrap, and store in the freezer until ready to serve.

Chocolate Muffins with Toasted Coconut

MAKES 9 MUFFINS

Prep time: 10 minutes
Cook time: 20 minutes

These rich dark chocolate muffins get an extra boost of flavor from the shredded coconut in the batter. The flaked coconut and sliced almonds sprinkled on top get nicely toasted as the muffins bake, making an attractive garnish.

5 MEDJOOL DATES (PITTED)

3 EGGS

3 TABLESPOONS HONEY

1 TABLESPOON COCONUT OIL, MELTED

½ TEASPOON VANILLA EXTRACT

¾ CUP ALMOND FLOUR

3 TABLESPOONS ARROWROOT POWDER

½ TEASPOON BAKING SODA

¼ TEASPOON SALT

3 TABLESPOONS UNSWEETENED COCOA POWDER

⅓ CUP UNSWEETENED SHREDDED COCONUT

⅓ CUP COCONUT FLAKES

⅓ CUP SLICED ALMONDS

1. Preheat the oven to 350°F. Line a standard muffin tin with nine paper liners.

2. In a food processor, combine the dates, eggs, honey, coconut oil, and vanilla, and pulse until smooth and well combined.

3. In a large mixing bowl, stir together the almond flour, arrowroot powder, baking soda, salt, cocoa powder, and shredded coconut. Add the egg mixture to the flour mixture and stir to mix well.

continued ▶

4. Spoon the batter into the prepared muffin tin, dividing it equally among the nine muffin cups. Top each muffin with a sprinkling of coconut flakes and almonds.

5. Bake for 20 minutes. Transfer the muffins to a wire rack to cool. Serve warm or at room temperature.

Chocolate Mug Cake

Prep time: 2 minutes
Cook time: 2 minutes

This is the perfect thing when you are struck with a sudden and uncontrolla-ble craving for something sweet and chocolaty. It literally takes less than five minutes to make. This handy recipe makes one serving—but is easily doubled or tripled, of course!

3 TABLESPOONS ALMOND FLOUR
3 TABLESPOONS COCOA POWDER
2 TABLESPOONS HONEY
1 TEASPOON VANILLA EXTRACT
1 EGG, LIGHTLY BEATEN
PINCH OF SALT
PINCH OF GROUND CINNAMON

1. Stir all ingredients together in a microwave-safe mug.

2. Microwave on high for 2 minutes. Serve hot.

Molten Chocolate Cakes

Prep time: 10 minutes
Cook time: 15 minutes

This decadent chocolate dessert contains a bit of coconut sugar, so it should be reserved for a special treat. It is so rich and satisfying that it is absolutely worth splurging on.

¼ CUP COCONUT OIL, PLUS MORE FOR THE RAMEKINS
1 TEASPOON COCONUT FLOUR, PLUS MORE FOR THE RAMEKINS
4 OUNCES DARK CHOCOLATE
2 EGGS
½ TEASPOON VANILLA EXTRACT
⅛ TEASPOON SALT
2 TABLESPOONS COCONUT PALM SUGAR
2 TEASPOONS COCOA POWDER

1. Preheat the oven to 375°F. Grease four 6-ounce ramekins with coconut oil, then dust the insides of the ramekins with a bit of coconut flour.

2. Place the chocolate and the ¼ cup of coconut oil in a 4-cup glass measuring cup with a spout, or in a medium microwave-safe bowl. Microwave on low in 30 second increments until the chocolate is mostly melted. Stir until smooth and set aside.

3. In a medium bowl, using an electric mixer, beat together the eggs, vanilla, salt, and coconut palm sugar until the mixture becomes frothy, about 5 minutes.

4. Add the egg mixture to the chocolate. Sift the cocoa powder and the 1 teaspoon coconut flour into the mixture and stir gently to combine.

5. Pour the batter into the prepared ramekins, dividing it equally (the batter should fill the ramekins with about ½ inch of space at the top). Place the filled ramekins on a baking sheet and bake for 12 minutes.

6. Let the ramekins cool on a rack for a few minutes, then invert the cakes onto small serving plates. Serve immediately.

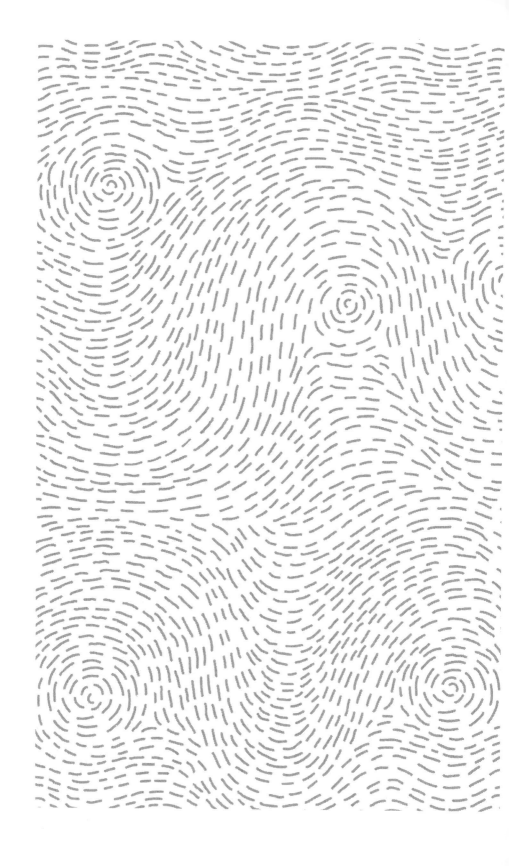

Resources

There are plenty of sources for information about the Paleo diet, Paleo-friendly recipes, and Paleo foods. Here are a few favorites.

BLOGS

Hunter-Gatherer
http://huntergatherer.com

Hunt. Gather. Love.
http://huntgatherlove.com

PALEO FOOD SOURCES

Amazon
Search the "Grocery" department for "Paleo," and you'll find all sorts of Paleo-friendly foods, including nut flours and healthy oils, granolas and snack bars, energy balls, baking mixes, coconut butter, and more.
www.amazon.com

Paleo People
http://www.paleopeople.com

Paleo Treats
http://www.paleotreats.com

Whole Foods
Whole Foods and other natural foods stores carry coconut oil, coconut butter, coconut flour, nut flours, nut butters, and other essentials of the well-rounded Paleo diet.
www.wholefoodsmarket.com

WEBSITES

Mark's Daily Apple
http://www.marksdailyapple.com

Paleo Plan
http://www.paleoplan.com

The Paleo Diet
http://thepaleodiet.com

Index

38711592R00086

Made in the USA
San Bernardino, CA
13 June 2019